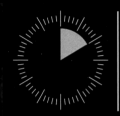

The 10-minute consultation:
persistent pain

Editors

Dr Martin Johnson
RCGP Clinical Lead for Chronic Pain

and

Dr Ann Taylor
School of Medicine
Cardiff University
UK

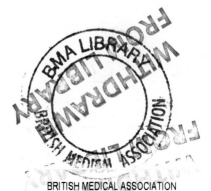

Published by Cedilla Publishing Limited

PO Box 58871, London SE15 9BE, UK

Telephone: +44 (0)7794 485294

www.cedillapublishing.com

The publisher and authors have made every effort to ensure the accuracy
of the information in this book, but cannot accept responsibility for any
errors or omissions. Any product mentioned in this publication should be
used in accordance with the local prescribing information prepared by
the manufacturers. No claims or endorsements are made for any drug or
compound at present under clinical investigation.

British Library Cataloguing in Publication Data

A catalogue for this book is available from the British Library.

ISBN: 978-1-905982-10-3

10 9 8 7 6 5 4 3 2 1

Printed by Ashford Colour Press in the UK.

Contents

Foreword   **v**
Maureen Baker

1. Introduction   **1**

Why *The 10-minute consultation: persistent pain*?   1
Martin Johnson

Aims and objective of the book   1
Ann Taylor

Epidemiology of persistent pain   2
Ceri Phillips

The nature of pain   4
Justin Taylor, Tony Dickenson, Irene Tracey, and Blair H. Smith

Legislation, legal and ethical issues   12
Kevin Markham

2. Assessment of the patient with pain   **14**

Overarching principles of pain assessment   14
Chris Barker and Becky Sim

Screening and assessment tools   20
Justin Taylor

3. How to manage the patient with persistent pain   **24**

Introduction to the principles of pain management   24
Martin Johnson, Jonathan Hill, Paul Watson, Owen Hughes, Roger Knaggs, Helen Radford, and Joan Hester

Management of chronic LBP and sciatica   48

Sanjeeva Gupta and Manohair Sharma

Chronic widespread pain and fibromyalgia   57

Benjamin Ellis

Pelvic pain   70

John Hughes

Neuropathic pain   79

Blair H. Smith and Mick Serpell

Managing co-morbidities   88

Amanda C de C Williams, Sarah Fox and Neil Stanley

4. Person-centred care   **114**

Self-management   114

Frances Cole

Principles of self-management   115

Frances Cole

What is a pain self-management programme?   120
   A simple guide for GPs and patients from
   a patient's perspective

Peter Moore

Further reading   **122**

Foreword

Persistent pain affects around 20% of our population and patients with persistent pain consult their general practitioner (GP) fives times more frequently than those without.

This useful handbook aims to raise awareness of persistent pain for those working in primary care and who manage the vast majority of cases.

It has been developed by experts – including GPs – in the field of persistent pain, with the following objectives:

- To explain the main elements of pathophysiology.
- To outline how to assess the patient with persistent pain and understand the biopsychosocial approach.
- To increase understanding of the range of treatments available, especially the importance of supported self-management and how drugs are not the only treatment option for persistent pain.

Helpful case studies are also included in a supplementary volume to support primary care professionals in understanding the complex web of multiple pain types and how they can be managed in primary care or referred appropriately.

An easy-to-use clinical guide that focusses on the initial assessment and management of pain for those who are not pain specialists is currently missing from the portfolio of resources available to health professionals. We hope that this book will fill the gap and that it will be used widely by GP trainees, as well as more senior practitioners, in caring for our patients who present with pain in primary care.

Dr Maureen Baker
Chair of Council
Royal College of General Practitioners

Chapter 1
Introduction

Why *The 10-minute consultation: persistent pain?*

Martin Johnson

How important are the accurate and timely assessment and subsequent management of persistent pain problems in primary care patients? "Worthwhile?", "Easy?" and "Time-consuming?" are some of the responses that I get when asking the same question in my lectures on persistent pain. Fundamentally, many healthcare professionals fail to realise what persistent pain is and also the burden it creates on society and the individual. It can be argued that persistent pain is the most common symptomatic long-term condition treated in primary care, and yet it is given one of the lowest priorities. General practice can be characterized as the art of unravelling the medically unexplained – this book is our attempt to help spread the word that primary care has a crucial role in the assessment and management of persistent pain. We are extremely grateful to all our authors for their expert contributions.

Aims and objectives of the book

Ann Taylor

The aim of this book is to provide primary care teams with a quick-reference guide to support effective, patient-centred and evidence-based pain management. Specifically, we have the following objectives:

- To justify why early and effective pain management is important, especially given that chronic non-malignant pain is a long-term condition in its own right.
- To ground pain within a biopsychosocial model.

- To provide pragmatic approaches to screen, assess, diagnose and manage pain.
- To align the management of commonly seen pain conditions to the British Pain Society's Pain Patient Map of Medicine Pathways and introduce case studies for consideration (supplementary resources are available in the ebook version).

Epidemiology of persistent pain

Ceri Phillips

A supplementary video is available in the ebook version or from the Pain Community Centre website.

The economics of pain | Ceri Phillips

⊙ http://www.paincommunitycentre.org/article/economics-pain

Time required: 60 minutes

- Persistent pain represents a major public health problem, having a larger negative impact on quality of life than any other chronic disorder for people living in the community (Table 1.1). It has a major impact on employment, interfering with the ability to work, and is associated with increased mortality, especially if those affected are unable to be active.

Impact of persistent pain	
Work	
Unemployment rates	Significantly higher
Disability	Significantly higher
Productivity	Significantly lower
Healthcare use	
GP visits	Significantly higher
Hospitalizations	Significantly higher
Quality of life	
Wellbeing	Significantly lower

Table 1.1 GP, general practitioner.

- Estimates of the prevalence of persistent pain vary, but it is reasonable to assume that, across the UK, one in three households contain an individual who is suffering with persistent pain, which translates to approximately one in eight people who live with a painful condition.

- Although some people learn to live reasonably well with their condition, others find it seriously affects their daily activities, as well as their social and working lives.

- Persistent pain has a larger negative impact on quality of life and wellbeing than other conditions and is associated with some of the poorest quality-of-life indices – for example:

  - 65% of people with persistent pain report difficulty sleeping.

  - Nearly 50% of people with persistent pain are depressed and have problems conducting social activities, walking, driving or having a normal sex life.

  - Over 40% of people with persistent pain report that it has a negative impact on family and friends.

  - More than 40% of people with persistent pain feel they have become socially isolated because of their pain.

- The extent of the persistent pain problem poses a significant economic burden for patients, health services and societies alike:

  - Those with persistent pain use healthcare services significantly more often than those without persistent pain.

  - People with persistent pain have more consultations with general practitioners (GPs), are more frequently hospitalized, spend more days in hospital and consume substantial quantities of medication compared with those without persistent pain.

- The economic impact of pain is greater than most other health conditions, because of increased rates of absenteeism, reduced levels of productivity and increased risks of people leaving the labour market and moving into long-term incapacity and disability, with enormous costs to employers and economies – constituting nearly 3% of the annual UK gross domestic product.

The nature of pain

Definitions of pain

Justin Taylor

The International Association for the Study of Pain defines 'pain' as follows:

> "… an unpleasant sensory and emotional experience associated with actual or potential tissue damage, or described in terms of such damage."

McCaffrey and Beebe (1989) offered an alternative definition:

> "Pain is whatever the experiencing person says it is, existing whenever the experiencing person say it does."

Both of these definitions highlight that a painful experience is more than just tissue damage that triggers a response from the nervous system. The management of pain thus involves more than simply treating the tissue injury.

So having defined pain, it is important to have a clear understanding of how acute pain differs from persistent pain:

* Acute pain is short-lasting, is a symptom, has an identifiable pathology as a response to tissue damage, has a biological function, is usually relieved by treatment and can be associated with anxiety.

* Persistent pain is long-lasting, has an often unidentifiable pathology as a response to unknown peripheral or central changes in the somatosensory cortex, has no biological function, can sometimes be unresponsive to treatment and can be associated with several emotional symptoms (eg, depression and feelings of hopelessness).

Although acute or 'nociceptive' pain is distinct from persistent pain, the boundaries are not always well-defined. Those with acute pain can suffer through more than one mechanism at a given time (ie, ischaemic, visceral, somatic, neuropathic or procedural pain). Furthermore, although acute pain has a foreseeable end, its management should be a high priority, because it can, if neglected, become chronic and persistent.

It is important to identify a neuropathic element in the acute pain history because management options differ for those experiencing neuropathic pain compared with those used for nociceptive pain. The following features in the acute pain history might suggest a neuropathic element:

* Clinical circumstances associated with a high risk of nerve injury – for example, thoracic or chest wall procedures, amputations or hernia repairs.
* Pain descriptors (Table 1.2).
* The paroxysmal or spontaneous nature of the pain, which might have no clear precipitating factors.

Assistive tool for determining types of acute pain			
	Somatic pain	**Visceral pain**	**Neuropathic pain**
Location	Localized	Generalized	Radiating or specific
Patient description	Pin prick, stabbing or sharp	Ache, pressure or sharp	Burning, pricking, tingling, electric shock or lancinating
Mechanism of pain	Delta-fibre activity in the periphery	C-fibre activity involving deeper innervation	Dermatomal (peripheral) or non-dermatomal (central)
Clinical examples	Superficial laceration, superficial burns, intramuscular injections, venous access, otitis media, stomatitis and extensive abrasions	Periosteum, joints, muscle injury, colic and muscle spasm, sickle cell crisis, appendicitis and kidney stones	Trigeminal neuralgia, post-traumatic neuralgia, peripheral neuropathy, post-herpetic neuralgia, complex regional pain syndrome and phantom limb pain

Table 1.2 Adapted from Institute for Clinical Systems Improvement: Assessment and Management of Acute Pain (2008). http://sonoranhealth.org/resources/Acute+Pain$2C+2008.pdf (accessed 7th March 2014).

- The presence of spontaneous or evoked unpleasant abnormal sensations (dysaesthesias).

- Increased response to abnormally painful stimulus (hyperalgesia).

- Pain owing to a stimulus that does not normally evoke pain (allodynia).

- Areas of numbness (hypoaesthesia).

- Changes in colour, temperature and sweating in the affected area and phantom phenomena.

Thus, when planning effective pain management, it is important to establish the pain mechanism involved (Table 1.2), in addition to considering the idiosyncrasies and needs of the specific patient group.

Pain physiology, mechanisms and sites of action

Tony Dickenson and Irene Tracey

Supplementary videos are available in the ebook version or from the Pain Community Centre website.

Advances on mechanisms of transition from acute to chronic pain | Tony Dickenson

⊙ http://www.paincommunitycentre.org/article/advances-mechanisms-transition-acute-chronic-pain

Time required: 30 minutes

Update on pain mechanisms | Tony Dickenson

⊙ http://www.paincommunitycentre.org/article/update-pain-mechanisms-tony-dickenson

Time required: 60 minutes

Imaging pain | Irene Tracey

⊙ http://www.paincommunitycentre.org/article/imaging-pain

Time required: 60 minutes

- The two broad, major types of persistent pain, neuropathic and inflammatory pain, involve both peripheral and central processes (Figure 1.1).

- Low back pain (LBP) and cancer pain can be either type of pain or, more often, a combination of both types. The peripheral mechanisms of these types of pain are different; yet, the signalling systems seem to be similar within the central nervous system.

- In pain conditions that are often called 'idiopathic' or 'dysfunctional', such as fibromyalgia and irritable bowel syndrome, the underlying mechanisms are more likely to be central than peripheral.

- Pain sensors in the periphery are likely to be continually activated when tissue is damaged, including ongoing production of inflammatory mediators – these can be modulated by local steroids or non-steroidal anti-inflammatory drugs (NSAIDs)/cyclo-oxygenase inhibitors.

- In neuropathic pain, changes in ion channels, in particular sodium channels, cause abnormal peripheral drives and marked changes in calcium channels occur in the spinal cord – carbamazepine and gabapentin/pregabalin suppress these activities.

- In the spinal cord, the release of transmitters activates receptors that generate central hypersensitivity/sensitization.

- Heightened messages to the sensory and emotional parts of the brain ensue and co-morbidities, such as depression, sleep disturbances and anxiety, are common.

- Messages from the brain can descend to facilitate/inhibit spinal mechanisms of nociceptive processing via the descending pain modulatory system: this 'top-down' influence directly controls what nociceptive inputs arrive in the brain and so powerfully controls the resultant pain experienced.

- This system allows a crucial interplay between sensory and psychological events in nociceptive processing and resultant pain perception. Opioids act at spinal and brain sites, and tricyclic antidepressants (TCAs)/serotonin–norepinephrine reuptake inhibitors (SNRIs) act to modulate these powerful descending controls, which fail in persistent pain states.

- In the brain, after extensive modulation from these top-down influences, arriving nociceptive inputs are routed to a flexibly accessible and extensive bilateral network of regions that

Pathways and processes in pain

Somatosensory cortex (via thalamic relays) *intensity and location of pain*

Persistent Pain

Potential re-organization

Amygdala *Fear, anxiety, aversion*

Persistent Pain

Ongoing and enhanced activity in affective centres

Genotype (eg, Na, TRPV1, etc) Individual sensory phenotype Prior pain experience Environmental factors Context Metabolic factors

Persistent Pain

Enhanced pain messages Co-morbidities – anxiety and depression Pain memories Altered descending controls

Autonomic changes Sleep disturbances

CC

PO

VPM/ VPL Hyp

PAG

PB

A7

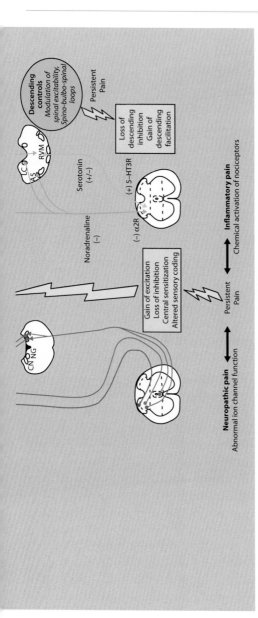

Figure 1.1 5-HT3R, 5-hydroxytryptamine receptor 3; [alpha symbol]2R, alpha-2 adrenoceptor; A5 and A7, cell bodies of noradrenaline neurones; Am, amygdala; CC, cerebral cortex; CN, cuneate nucleus; Hyp, hypothalamus; LC, locus coeruleus; Na, sodium; NG, nucleus gracilis; PAG, periaqueductal grey; PB, parabrachial nucleus; Po, posterior thalamus; RVM, rostroventral medial medulla; TRPVI, transient receptor potential vanilloid 1; VPL, ventral posterior lateral nucleus of the thalamus; VPM, ventral posterior medial nucleus of the thalamus. The figure depicts the various ascending pathways from the spinal cord to the brain on the left and the descending pathways from the brain back to the spinal cord on the right. For further details, see D'Mello R and Dickenson AH (2008) Spinal cord mechanisms of pain. *Br J Anaesth* **101**:8–16.

encode key features of the multidimensional experience that is 'pain' – for example:

- Sensory location and intensity.
- Unpleasantness and threat/fear.
- Attention and decision-making.
- Movement and memory.
- If the patient's current mood, cognitive state or expectancy or the context of their environment changes, this network is flexibly accessed, even to the same nociceptive input from the damaged area of the body, and produces a change in the pain experienced.
- Pain is a highly malleable perception that can be powerfully modulated by increasingly well-understood brain networks because of these various factors.
- Various centrally acting pharmacological agents are increasingly recognised as influencing these brain circuits, and it is likely that cognitive-behavioural therapies mediate their effects by changing these dynamic networks.

The biopsychosocial nature of pain

Justin Taylor

- The biomedical model considers pain to have a solely biological origin and be explained solely in medical terms and has been used traditionally as the basis of medical diagnosis and management.
- The biomedical model acknowledges that mental or emotional problems might be the end result of having persistent pain but maintains that the pain itself is biological in origin.
- Medical approaches are the only successful treatment for persistent pain proposed under the biomedical model.
- Persistent pain and disability cannot be explained purely in terms of physical disease, however, because structural lesions that account for the person's pain cannot always be identified.
- The biomedical model also fails to explain why different people with the same physical injury or disease respond to it so differently.
- Biological, psychological and social factors should be considered for a more complete understanding of pain:

- 'Psychological' factors are the mental, emotional and behavioural aspects of pain.
- 'Social' factors are interactions with other people.
- According to the biopsychosocial model, it is impossible to fully understand the problem of pain using physical or medical concepts alone, both the mind and the body are considered inextricably linked.
- One negative way in which these elements often overlap is in the creation of a vicious circle of pain (p. 115) – for example:
  - Pain sensations (sensory) often result in decreased physical activity (actions).
  - Decreased physical activity can create feelings of depression (emotional) and decreased self-worth (mental).
  - Depression can lead to decreased motivation and even less activity (actions).
  - Decreased activity, accompanied by withdrawal from other people (social), leads to even more depression, preoccupation with negative thoughts (mental) and increased awareness of pain.
- Although clinicians cannot always control patients' pain sensations and negative emotional reactions, they can usefully target the way in which a patient thinks and acts – this is the basis behind many talking therapies.

Risk factors for persistent pain

Blair H. Smith

- Risk factors for persistent pain include those for specific pain-related diagnoses (eg, diabetes, arthritis, back pain and surgical procedures).
- Independent sociodemographic risk factors for persistent pain include older age, female gender, manual occupation, lower education and social deprivation.
- Psychosocial risk factors include anxiety, depression, patients reporting with multiple physical symptoms and particular healthcare-consulting behaviours.

- The biggest risk is indeed pain itself, either an acute pain episode or a history of persistent pain(s) – most people with persistent pain will experience this at more than one site.

- Some risk factors are mainly identified by cross-sectional studies, and it is difficult to distinguish cause from effect – there is often a 'bidirectional' aetiology (eg, persistent pain leads to depression, and vice versa).

- Other risk factors (eg, age and gender) are non-modifiable but inform targeting of treatment and prevention.

- Further research is required into the biological mechanisms behind these risks, to inform prevention – for example, the stress response, via the hypothalamo–pituitary–adrenal axis, and genetic factors.

- The identification of risk factors is likely to have an increasingly important role in primary care in ensuring early detection and management of potential/actual chronicity.

Legislation, legal and ethical issues

Kevin Markham

- The relief of pain is a core ethical duty in healthcare, and in 2010 representatives from 129 countries supported a declaration that access to pain management is a fundamental human right (Montréal Declaration):

"No one should be subject … to inhuman or degrading treatment."

Article 5 of the Universal Declaration of Human Rights

- In several US states, statutory rights exist for pain relief, which means obligatory referral to a pain physician – in the absence of legislation, constitutional rights, such as those espoused in the US Constitution, provide support for the alleviation of pain.

- There is little UK or European legislation governing pain, so ethical considerations provide the way forward.

- Evidence-based guidelines, in general, have enhanced the quality and safety of practice for both patients and health professionals.

- Adherence to guidelines can provide a more favourable outcome in litigation – non-adherence is acceptable, providing it is supported by rational argument.

- In the US, pain is recognised as 'an injury at law', a legal entity – litigation for negligence arises from three main causes:
  - Under-treatment of pain.
  - Over-treatment of pain.
  - Failure to diagnose.

- Compensated claims for injury sustained during pain-relief procedures are rare.

Overarching principles of pain assessment

Chris Barker and Becky Sim

A supplementary video is available in the ebook version or from the Pain Community Centre website.

Assessing chronic pain in the GP time-slice | Chris Barker

▶http://www.paincommunitycentre.org/article/assessing-chronic-pain-gp-time-slice

Time required: 20 minutes

Keywords

- Biopsychosocial.
- Diagnosis.
- Understanding.
- Agreement.
- Management.

Objectives

- To assess biological, psychological and functional factors quickly and accurately.
- To develop a working diagnosis(es).
- To effectively identify important medical conditions that cause or contribute to the overall pain state.
- To mutually agree on an effective management plan (the person living with pain and the clinician).

- To recognise when complex problems exist and the need for more in-depth assessment and management (and potentially an onward referral).

Background

- Accurate pain assessment underpins all aspects of pain management. For treatment to be effective, it is necessary to have a good understanding of the problem. This is true of new pain presentations or repeated, refractory ones.

- The assessment of any new pain is often taken up by making a diagnosis, but it is easy to ignore the assessment of the pain itself and also psychosocial issues, which are often highly relevant.

- Serious pathology must be ruled out, but initially this approach could take the focus away from the presenting pain that requires explanation. It is important to share this with the patient from the outset.

- The clinical skill is in balancing the agreement of priorities, ensuring patient safety and agreeing effective management.

- Primary care clinicians have the essential role of initially being aware of the possibility of a diagnosis of persistent pain, and then helping the patient onto the correct treatment pathway by performing the vital first assessment.

Screening

- Because of time constraints for the consultation, screening might help the clinician decide on how to approach the assessment of a patient presenting with pain.

- Initial screening tools can inform what needs to happen at the initial and subsequent consultations and are important for the following reasons:

  - Identification of significant illness is important at an early stage.

  - The presence of 'red flags' is an indicator for either further investigation or urgent referral.

- • Other symptoms and signs are taken on merit and can either be investigated in primary care or be referred on urgently, depending on severity.
- Psychosocial barriers to recovery are extremely important and, if present, require more in-depth assessment and management.
- Further screening and assessment might be required if either of the two following questions elicits a positive response:

  1. In the past month, has your pain been bad enough to often make you feel worried or low in mood?

  2. In the past month, has your pain been bad enough to often make you unable to carry out your day to day activities?

- Psychosocial barriers to recovery ('yellow flags'; Table 2.1) are prognostic indicators that highlight risk for the development of chronicity, and there is good evidence to support early intervention to prevent this.
- Recognition of yellow flags in the consultation is important; however, acting on their presence is less easy. It might require additional time individually with patients or recognising that referral might be the best course of action.

Assessment

Pain assessment has three fundamental 'pillars':

- Biological:
  - Diagnosis.

Examples of yellow flags
• Belief that persistent pain is harmful or disabling
• Fear-avoidant behaviour
• Tendency to low mood and social withdrawal
• Expectation of benefit from passive treatments

Table 2.1

- The what, where, when and how of pain.
- Pain intensity, nature and character.
- Psychological – distress, for example in the form of the following:
  - Fear.
  - Depression.
  - Anxiety.
  - Catastrophizing.
  - Unhelpful heath beliefs.
  - Impact of loss on the person.
  - Having to navigate life in a different way than before.
  - Aberrant drug use.
- Social (or functional):
  - Disability.
  - Relationships with family, friends, work and society.

All the 'pillars' are needed to construct an accurate assessment of pain, and each has equal merit. Knowledge of the three pillars leads to a working diagnosis, which can be shared with the patient, and so an agreed management plan can be formulated.

The following section identifies the important components to consider for each pillar.

Biological

- Ensure patient safety (early establishment of red flags – serious pathology).
- Identify the need for further investigations or urgent opinions.
- Pain – onset, duration and exacerbating or relieving factors.
- Previous and present treatment(s).
- Appropriate clinical examination.
- Establishing a working diagnosis(es).

Psychological

- Understanding distress (either pain-related or not).
- Evaluating health beliefs:

- Fear is a potent predictor of disability.
- Psychological distress is a potent risk for chronicity of pain and disability.
- Pain is exacerbated by distress.
- Catastrophizing can lead to worry and anxiety, and further exacerbate fear.

Social

- Understanding functionality:
  - Individually.
  - Within the family.
  - Within the workplace.
  - Socially.

General points in the assessment consultation

- A real understanding of patient issues helps inform the assessment.
- An empathetic approach is important; often, patients have 'good reasons' for behaving as they do. It is crucial that the patient feels listened to and believed; indeed, remember that many patients with persistent pain have had poor experiences of previous health care.
- Complex problems need more than 10 minutes – it might be necessary to arrange further assessment in a future appointment (or double appointment).
- It is often impossible to cover all the agendas that the patient presents with. This can be helped by openness with the patient and sharing the dilemma – for example:
  - "We have 10 minutes left today. I have to ask a bit more about your pain to ensure nothing serious has been missed and then we can focus on some of the things you mentioned like medicines, injections or how the pain is affecting you. Which do you want to focus on?"
  - "To do this justice, we won't be able to cover everything today but can make another time to think further … ."

- Use joint working to establish the patient's needs and expectations – for example:

  - The patient will often say "I want to get rid of this pain!", which is often not easily achievable (if at all).

  - 'Getting rid of this pain' can be broken down into smaller, more manageable components and these need exploring.

- Understand concerns by listening actively:

  - Summarize what the patient says.

  - Ask the patient if you have understood them correctly.

  - Maintain eye contact.

Diagnosis

It is uncommon in established persistent pain for there only to be one unifying diagnosis. Multiple diagnoses *per se* are not necessarily problematic if managed appropriately. The concept of different aetiologies responsible for different aspects of pain is a useful one in rehabilitation. This can enable specific management of each one without confusion. It highlights the importance of an agreed management plan (with the aim of working to meaningful goals set by the patient), which runs concurrently with the establishment of a diagnosis and is a constant the patient can refer to. Even in situations in which the diagnosis might not be clear-cut, there are many useful strategies that can be employed to preserve functionality and maximize wellbeing:

- A working diagnosis is important in the management of pain, but this should be considered equal in importance to agreed effective management of pain.

- Ensure that there is consistency in diagnosis – persistent pain sufferers often have been given many differing diagnoses by different clinicians (in addition to their own perceived ones).

- Clinicians might have used a variety of terms to explain the same thing but patients perceive them as different diagnoses – for example, "Dr, I have osteoarthritis, degenerative disease, and wear and tear!"

- Patients often remember the first diagnosis they are told, which is why correct assessment in primary care is vital.
- Ageing is not a disease.

Role of the GP

- Do believe the patient.
- Do recognise when to medicalize.
- Do listen carefully for the 'real problem'.
- Do facilitate a shared approach to diagnosis and management (collaborate with the patient).
- Do co-ordinate the patient's care.
- Do facilitate the patient's ownership of their problem and allow them responsibility for change.
- Don't ignore the patient's expertise in managing their problem (instead notice and compliment their strengths).
- Don't unilaterally decide the management plan (including simply switching/increasing analgesics).
- Don't medicalize when not needed.
- Don't scare with medical jargon or catastrophic speak (eg, 'crumbling bones').
- Don't disempower patient decision-making.

Screening and assessment tools

Justin Taylor

A supplementary video is available in the ebook version or from the Pain Community Centre website.

Assessment of neuropathic pain | Mike Bennett

▶ http://www.paincommunitycentre.org/article/assessment-neuropathic-pain

Time required: 20 minutes

Satisfactory treatment is only possible after a comprehensive assessment of not only the biological aetiology of the pain, but also the patient's psychosocial and behavioural presentation, including their emotional state (anxiety, depression and anger), perception and understanding of their symptoms, and the reactions to those symptoms by significant others (p. 9).

Apart from a well-conducted physical examination and history-taking, a brief screening interview (or questionnaire) might be used initially, followed by a more in-depth interview or questionnaire(s), depending on the responses provided. Although there is nothing new about using screening questionnaires to complement history-taking, the use of these measurements to guide diagnosis and treatment, at first presentation and to assess treatment outcomes, is gaining momentum. The benefit of screening is that it alerts clinicians much earlier to co-existing conditions that might affect outcomes and treatment failures, which can in turn 'ramp up' the associated frustration that patients and practitioners inevitably feel. Using this systematic and structured approach is pivotal for successful patient self-management, primary and specialty clinical care, and determining the quality of an individual or group practice. Using this strategy also helps define key determinants for stepping up treatment by introducing other multimodal treatment options.

With limited time available, a unidimensional self-report measure is commonly used:

- A numerical rating scale that asks the patient to "Rate your typical pain on a scale from 0 to 10, where 0 equals 'no pain' and 10 is pain 'as bad as it could be'."

- A verbal rating scale that asks the patient "Is your usual level of pain 'mild', 'moderate' or 'severe'?"

Another useful tool consists of a two-item pain intensity and interference scale (Figure 2.1). Its main use is in the assessment of opioid treatment, in terms of pain intensity and physical function.

Two examples of brief psychological screening tools use the acronym 'ACT-UP' (Activity, Coping, Think, Upset, People's responses; Tables 2.2 and 2.3). A positive response to any of the questions in either of these pre-screening tools should prompt further questioning by the clinician or a more detailed evaluation.

Two-question pain intensity and interference measure

1. **In the last month**, on average, how would you rate your pain? Rate your typical pain on a scale from 0 to 10, where 0 equals 'no pain' and 10 is pain 'as bad as it could be'.

No pain   **As bad as it could be**

0	1	2	3	4	5	6	7	8	9	10

2. **In the last month**, how much has pain interfered with your daily activities? Use a scale from 0 to 10, where 0 is 'no interference' and 10 is 'unable to carry on any activities'.

No interference   **Unable to carry on any activities**

0	1	2	3	4	5	6	7	8	9	10

Figure 2.1 Developed by Von Korff M *et al.* and adapted from Washington State Agency Medical Directors' Group (2010) Interagency Guideline on Opioid Dosing for Chronic Non-Cancer Pain: an Educational Aid to Improve Care and Safety with Opioid Treatment. http://www.agencymeddirectors.wa.gov/Files/OpioidGdline.pdf (accessed 14th August 2014).

ACT-UP psychological screening tool

1. **A**ctivity: how is your pain affecting your life (ie, sleep, appetite, physical activities and relationships)?

2. **C**oping: how do you deal/cope with your pain (what makes it better/worse)?

3. **T**hink: do you think your pain will ever get better?

4. **U**pset: have you been feeling worried (anxious) or depressed (down or blue)?

5. **P**eople: how do people respond to you when you have pain?

Table 2.2 Adapted from Dansie EJ and Turk DC (2013) Assessment of patients with chronic pain. *Br J Anaesth* **111**:19–25.

Serious depression and anxiety often exist in tandem with persistent pain, with an estimated prevalence of >50%. Measuring mood at each clinical encounter could be considered essential. The nine-question Patient Health Questionnaire (PHQ-9) is an effective questionnaire to measure and monitor patient mood. The seven-question General Anxiety and Depression Instrument (GAD-7) can be used similarly to monitor anxiety.

Short pre-screening assessment	
Ask the following two questions	
1. Over the past 2 weeks, has pain been bad enough to interfere with your day-to-day activities?	
2. Over the past 2 weeks, have you felt worried or low in mood because of this pain?	
Evaluate	
• Pain duration	'… past 2 weeks …'
• Pain intensity	'… pain been bad enough …'
• Level of pain-related disability	'… day-to-day activities …'
• Level of pain-related distress	'… worried or low in mood …'

Table 2.3 Developed by one of the contributing authors of this book and adapted from Barker C *et al.* (2014) Problematic pain – redefining how we view pain? *Br J Pain* **8:**9–15.

This section does not aim to cover the myriad of psychological and behavioural questionnaires that are available but offers several 'ways in' for primary care practitioners to quickly and easily access and respond to changes in pain, physical function, depression and anxiety. Further discussion on the areas raised by the questionnaires or referral for a multiprofessional evaluation can be tailored by either cut-off scores or a rising trend in scores.

The Initial Assessment and Early Management Pathway of the British Pain Society's Pain Patient Map of Medicine Pathways provides further guidance and tools for screening and assessing pain.

Chapter 3

How to manage the patient with persistent pain

Introduction to the principles of pain management

Martin Johnson, Jonathan Hill, Paul Watson, Owen Hughes, Roger Knaggs, Helen Radford and Joan Hester

It is important to recognise that patients with persistent pain often revolve around the healthcare system for many years, with either themselves and/or their healthcare professionals seeking the elusive 'cure' for their long-term condition of pain. This would not happen for any other long-term condition. The following chapter outlines many of the basic principles of managing persistent pain in a community setting.

Non-drug management

Supplementary videos are available in the ebook version or from the Pain Community Centre website.

Patient consultation with a psychologist: Case study 1 | Owen Hughes

⦿ http://www.paincommunitycentre.org/article/patient-consultation-psychologist-case-study-1

Time required: 20 minutes

Patient consultation with a psychologist: Case study 2 | Owen Hughes

⦿ http://www.paincommunitycentre.org/article/patient-consultation-psychologist-case-study-2

Time required: 20 minutes

Patient consultation with a psychologist: Case study 3 | Owen Hughes

⊙http://www.paincommunitycentre.org/article/patient-consultation-psychologist-case-study-3

Time required: 20 minutes

Keywords

- Disability.
- Psychosocial factors.
- Physical and psychological therapies.
- Functional rehabilitation.

Objectives

- To prevent further chronicity and the development of pain cycles by focussing on aspects contributing to an individual's ongoing pain experience – this is the primary aim of management.
- To keep the assessment and management approach broad – it might be necessary to start with medical aspects, but ensure the wider context is not overlooked.
- To be pro-active in motivating the individual to identify opportunities to improve wellbeing and function, often despite persistent ongoing pain.
- To actively agree realistic targets, including review appointments and monitoring of progress.

Background

- Pain is always 'in the brain', no matter how it starts, how long it persists or how it feels (sharp, strong, weak or mild). For this reason, biological, psychological, cultural, social and environmental factors all contribute to making the experience of living with pain unique to the individual; it is the brain that amalgamates all this information, leading to the pain experience.
- However, common risk factors for persistent pain have been identified, which can shed light on an individual's particular situation and should, therefore, be considered during assessment (Table 3.1).

Risk factors for persistent disability and pain

- High levels of co-morbidity (poor general health)
- Unhelpful illness beliefs and behaviours (eg, fearful of physical activity)
- Exaggerated perceived threat of pain (eg, pain is always demanding attention)
- Lack of control over symptoms (eg, poor individual ability to influence the pain)
- High levels of emotional impact from pain (eg, frequently bothered by the pain)
- Lack of hope related to future health (eg, pessimistic outlook of continued symptoms)
- Low/negative feeling and mood (eg, signs of social withdrawal or lack of motivation)
- Treatment inconsistent with best practice (eg, long-term strong opioids, passive or alarmist)
- Activity-avoidant behaviours (eg, extended bed rest or loss of daily routine)
- History of extended time off work or school/college
- Unhappy at work or employment disputes
- Ongoing medico-legal/ insurance claims
- Manual work with heavy lifting or working long and unsociable hours
- Lack of social support or an overprotective family

Table 3.1

Management

What questions to ask to inform management approaches?

Not all patients are overwhelmed or distressed by their persistent pain. An initial screen of the impact of symptoms on the individual can be useful to decide the extent to which clinical attention is required. If a patient is struggling, the clinician's time is invaluable; this is when it might be appropriate to use the two screening questions (p. 14).

If a more detailed assessment seems appropriate, it can be easy to overlook key pieces of the jigsaw, unless a structured assessment prompt is used, such as the one given in Table 3.2.

Structured assessment for persistent pain management

Establish the reason for the consultation

- Why has the individual come for this consultation today?
- How many times have they consulted already for this problem?
- What treatment have they had before?

Impact from symptoms (including work or family roles, if appropriate)

- What key activities and roles are they prevented from enjoying?
- What about interference from the pain on work or family roles? Remember that most musculoskeletal problems can be accommodated at work once obstacles have been identified and suggested workplace modifications are agreed. It is good to disclose that the practice will keep a record of an agreed return to work date
- Use fit notes to communicate with employers and encourage the patient to keep in touch with work

Medical action/referral

- Do they want or need a referral to a specialist, therapist or pain management team for support?
- Is medical action needed for potentially treatable pathology?

Pain control

- Is their current medication appropriate or having any adverse side effects?
- Do they feel sufficiently able to keep symptoms under control? What, apart from medication, is helpful?
- Consider autonomous use of painkillers, physical remedies and preventative adaptations/aids

Legitimization and education

- Has the cause of symptoms been properly explained?
- Do they know their likely prognosis?
- Have they got an ongoing plan for dealing with the symptoms?
- Are they healthcare literate and realistic about investigations?

Table 3.2

Opportunities for action

- Are there specific things that need to be done to help their confidence?

- Have they reflected on opportunities to keep active and healthy? For example, taking a leisurely stroll with friends, enjoying time with family and friends, being productive with a project, learning new skills, switching off from stress or finding others to share their story (perhaps online)?

- Is boredom an issue (eg, from being off work or unable to meet up with friends)?

- Do they have a daily routine?

- What down time/rests are they having during the day?

- How often are they prevented from doing things that are important to them?

- How are others responding to their pain (employer, co-workers and family)?

- Have they expressed the perception of being negatively judged for having persistent pain or that the impact of their pain is not taken seriously?

- Do they need to make adjustments to their role, identity and personal expectations? Some appropriate acceptance can often improve function. However, this might require a willingness to 'risk' further episodes in order to recover 'lost' activities or fulfil certain personal aspirations

- What was going on in their life around the time when the pain developed?

- Are there any useful links they can make themselves between a difficult time of life (relationships, finance and work) and a non-resolving pain picture? Recognising these links and improving self-awareness can be part of the healing process

- Are there issues with substance abuse or other unhealthy coping mechanisms?

Closure

- Is there anything else they would like to discuss?

- Do decisions need to be shared with others?

- Has there been an agreement about what follow-up is necessary/ appropriate and with whom?

Table 3.2 Continued.

Non-drug treatment targets

Review each of the following, with the evidence base from systematic review/meta-analytical studies:

- Functional rehabilitation.

- Psychological approaches (eg, cognitive-behavioural therapy, counselling, acceptance and commitment therapy, and mindfulness).

- Multidisciplinary management approaches (eg, pain management programmes).

- Interventional techniques (eg, transcutaneous electrical nerve stimulation [TENS], acupuncture and manipulations).

- Social support and third-sector organizations.

Role of the GP

Supplementary resources are available in the ebook version or from the Pain Community Centre website.

Pain toolkits

☞ http://www.paincommunitycentre.org/pain-toolkits

- Understanding the individual's unique needs is important for appropriately tailoring a management plan for someone in persistent pain. Some patients will need their symptoms legitimized and explained more than others, and it can be helpful to support your advice and reassurance with printed or online information (p. 116).

- Although it might be necessary to start with medical aspects of treatment, try to ensure that the wider context is not overlooked and the individual is fully engaged.

- Remember that a broad range of factors might be involved in contributing to an individual's ongoing pain experience and so several different aspects might need to be addressed simultaneously.

- Look for opportunities for action, using goals agreed with the patient that facilitate a healthy lifestyle and enhance as positive an outlook as possible, despite the pain (Table 3.2).

- Consider booking review appointments if you can, to re-iterate positive messages, encourage appropriate levels of activity, address misconceptions and monitor the patient's progress.
- Use a long-term condition approach for persistent pain, whereby the individual is supported to maintain their independence and self-manage their symptoms, as appropriate.

Options for referral

It is important to avoiding unnecessary, excessive or inappropriate treatment/investigation. However, appropriately provided conservative treatment can be a relatively cost-effective option, especially if clear expected outcomes are established at the start of treatment. Unfortunately, many patients are given unrealistic expectations before referral. Potential referral options are as follows:

- Consider physical therapies if pain and function are issues.
- Consider psychological expertise, if required, to ensure progress.
- Occupational rehabilitation.
- Pain clinics.
- Consider the use of local resources to help support self-management, such as expert patient programmes, walking groups or swimming groups.

Drug management

Keywords

- Drug management.
- Improving concordance.

Objectives

- To ensure pharmacological treatments for pain are prescribed within a biopsychosocial framework.
- To ensure treatment is individualized for each patient.
- To agree goals of treatment and discuss the benefits and potential side effects before prescribing.
- To consider rational polypharmacy, as appropriate.

Background

Medication is only one method of analgesia and should not be the sole focus of treatment for patients or healthcare professionals. Analgesics are most effective if used in conjunction with other treatment modalities to meet the overall treatment goals:

- A biopsychosocial approach to the patient is essential.
- Explore the use of other non-pharmacological methods (eg, self-management strategies or physiotherapy) with patients.
- The principles of the World Health Organization (WHO) analgesic ladder might be a useful starting point in a step-wise approach to management of inflammatory pain (Figure 3.1) but it should be remembered that it was intended originally for use in cancer pain and hence it should not be followed rigidly.
- Over-reliance on medication can be misplaced and unhelpful to the patient.

Management

Appropriate medication could include treatments for specific types of pain or adjunct therapies to treat co-morbidities such as depression and anxiety. Direct the use of medications not only toward

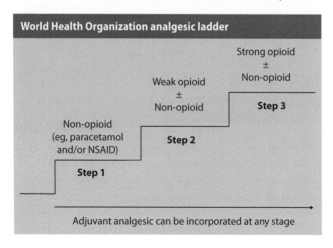

Figure 3.1 NSAID, non-steroidal anti-inflammatory drug.

pain relief, but also to increase physical, psychological and social functioning:

- If possible, identify the type of pain and treat any underlying cause (eg, better diabetes management should minimize the complications of diabetes, including pain) – base the initial choice of medication on the likely cause of pain.

- Patient factors (age, co-existing diseases, other medications and responses to previous treatments) can influence the likely response – discuss concordance with previous medications.

- Discuss likely benefits and possible side effects or risks of potential medications, particularly possible side effects.

- Agree the goals of treatment with each patient before prescribing, and adjust the choice of medications to meet his or her needs.

- Give each medication an adequate therapeutic trial and agree this period with the patient before initiating further treatment. Many analgesics require dose titration over several weeks and benefits can take several weeks to develop.

- Consider rational polypharmacy – appropriate use of analgesic combinations might produce improved efficacy and fewer adverse effects, because lower doses of individual medications are required.

- Avoid prescribing two drugs in the same class at the same time.

Treatment targets

Examples of appropriate drug treatments for specific types of pain are provided in Table 3.3.

Options

- Paracetamol is an effective analgesic, particularly for mild-to-moderate musculoskeletal pain, and is well-tolerated. While updating their guidance on the management of osteoarthritis, the National Institute for Clinical Excellence (NICE) highlighted new evidence that raises concerns about the long-term effectiveness and safety of paracetamol. As a consequence, the Medicines and Healthcare products

Condition-specific drug management

Target group	Suggested analgesia	Estimated timescale	Outcome
Simple mechanical low back pain	Paracetamol and/or NSAID	If pain is not resolving after 3 days, consider a 7-day course	Pain resolving and patient mobilizing
Post-herpetic neuralgia	Commence treatment with amitriptyline or gabapentin, or consider topical treatment if intolerant (eg, lignocaine 5% medicated plaster)	Patient needs to be aware that dose escalation might be required and optimal analgesia could take several weeks to develop	Pain relief acceptable Tolerable side effects
Osteoarthritis	Ibuprofen or naproxen is preferred first-line NSAID Consider the need for a PPI	Review prescribing after 1 month Regular review for efficacy and tolerability	Pain relief acceptable Tolerable side effects

Table 3.3 PPI, proton-pump inhibitor; NSAID, non-steroidal anti-inflammatory drug.

Regulatory Agency (MHRA) is currently reviewing the safety and over-the-counter (OTC) availability of NSAIDs and paracetamol. When this work is completed, NICE intends to commission a full update of the pharmacological management of osteoarthritis.

- Although NSAIDs are effective analgesics, their side effects must be monitored closely.

- Antidepressants and anti-epileptics are most effective in neuropathic pain.

- Use opioids with caution in non-cancer pain.

Role of the GP

- Select an appropriate medicine on the basis of the properties of the agent (onset, duration, available routes of administration, dosing intervals and side effects). This choice might also be affected by local and national guidelines (which will also take into consideration cost-effectiveness).
- Titrate doses to achieve the optimal balance between analgesic benefit, side effects and functional improvement.
- Optimize administration of analgesics. Generally, better pain control is obtained with regularly scheduled doses.
- Regularly review medicines for pain, including the four 'A's (p. 64):
  - Analgesia.
  - Adverse effects.
  - Activity (function of the patient).
  - Adherence.
- Taper and discontinue drugs that don't meet treatment goals.

Opioids

Keywords

- Opioids.
- Opioid trial.
- Side effects.
- Diversion.

Objectives

- To identify whether opioids are effective and safe for the management of persistent pain.
- To discuss how to select appropriate patients in whom to prescribe opioids.
- To present how to assess risk factors for possible misuse.
- To describe how to perform a trial of opioids.
- To explain how to choose an opioid.

- To discuss the monitoring of the patient taking long-term opioids.
- To identify when patients should be referred to a specialist.

Background

- Opioids are used effectively to treat severe acute pain, especially following trauma, and for pain associated with terminal illness.

- Opioids are also widely used in the management of chronic non-malignant pain, but this role is controversial because recent evidence indicates limited effectiveness and possible harms, including tolerance, dependency, addiction, reduced immunity to infection, endocrine effects and impaired cognitive function.

- There has been an exponential rise in the number of opioid prescriptions in primary care over the past 10 years.

- Mortality in the US from prescribed opioids for non-malignant pain is now greater than that from both suicide and road traffic accidents or deaths from cocaine and heroin combined, usually from accidental overdose in combination with other substances.

- There is a lack of detailed knowledge about opioids among non-pain-specialist healthcare professionals, including knowledge of pharmacokinetics, long-term side effects, equivalent doses, assessment of risk factors, monitoring and withdrawal.

- There is a perception that opioids are safe and effective, as often seems to be the case in the management of cancer pain, although the same problems with long-term use apply to cancer survivors.

Management

Safe and effective use of opioids for persistent pain

Don't use opioids as first-line therapy for chronic non-malignant pain. Use all other evidence-based pain management techniques first, for example self-management (including graded exercise, pacing and goal-setting), psychological therapies, TENS, acupuncture, simple injections and other appropriate medications.

There is no difference between short- and long-acting opioids with regard to effectiveness and long-term effects. Use the smallest possible dose for the shortest possible length of time. Recent evidence suggests that using small doses of a short-acting opioid in selected patients on an 'as-needed' basis can improve pain control, lower overall dosage and minimize adverse effects, contrary to the recommended use of opioids in palliative care. However, it is vital to follow prescribing and monitoring guidelines (p. 38).

The classification of opioids into 'strong' and 'weak' types is unhelpful, because so-called 'weak' opioids (codeine, dihydrocodeine and meptazinol) can have the same adverse effects as 'strong' opioids if used over a long period of time or in doses exceeding those recommended in the *British National Formulary* (*BNF*) or local guidelines. Tramadol is now classified by the *BNF* as a strong opioid.

Always initiate a trial of opioids before contemplating long-term use, with prior explanation of possible long-term effects and an agreement that the opioid will be withdrawn if the set goals are not achieved. In some countries (eg, the US and Denmark), a written contract is recommended between prescribers and selected patients before initiating long-term opioids, which might include a timeframe for visits to the doctor, a designated sole prescriber, use of short-term prescriptions and urine testing for breakdown products of opioids and other substances. At the present time, this is not suggested as standard practice in the UK but could be considered for an 'at-risk' patient (p. 36).

Consider the following before initiating opioids:

- What is the cause (diagnosis) of persistent pain in the patient?
- Opioids might be ineffective, hazardous or harmful in some pain conditions (Table 3.4).
- Has a full biopsychosocial assessment of the patient been made?
- Have any psychological issues been addressed, in particular anxiety and depression?

Conditions in which opioids are not recommended
• Sleep apnoea
• Headache
• Non-specific low back pain
• Fibromyalgia
• Unexplained persistent pain

Table 3.4

- Opioids relieve anxiety and it can be difficult to withdraw from them if they are used for this purpose – careful initial assessment is essential.

- Have other appropriate methods of pain management been tried? For example, self-management skills, graded exercises, psychological therapies, gabapentin and amitriptyline.

- Are risk factors for possible problem use of opioids present? If so, are they low, medium or high risk factors (p. 36)?

- There are risk-assessment questionnaires available – for example, The Screener and Opioid Assessment for Patients in Pain, revised 2007 (SOAPP-R).

- Will benefits outweigh possible harms in this particular patient? Take the necessary steps to define the answer to this question with your patient, who must be fully informed of benefits and risks and must agree to a trial of opioids, with possible withdrawal if it is ineffective. Table 3.5 illustrates in which groups opioids might be useful.

- Management of potential common side effects – for example, nausea, constipation and sedation.

Risk factors

Prescribe opioids with caution and an increased level of monitoring in certain patients (Table 3.6).

It is essential to perform a trial of opioids over a period not exceeding 6 weeks and withdraw them if agreed goals are not achieved (p. 38).

Conditions in which opioids might be appropriate
• Acute pain (trauma, heart attack and acute abdominal emergency)
• Cancer pain
• Sickle cell disease
• Neuropathic pain – eg, post-herpetic neuralgia, central post-stroke pain and post-surgical pain
• Visceral pain, with a well-defined cause – eg, pancreatitis and adhesions
• Severe arthritis

Table 3.5

Risk factors for the prescribing of opioids
• Age <45 years
• Mental health disorders
• Depression and/or anxiety related to pain
• Previous or existing inappropriate use, addiction or misuse of any substance, including diversion
• Concomitant use of drugs that depress the central nervous system, for example benzodiazepines and alcohol
• Serious mental health issues or addiction in the family

Table 3.6 One factor = low risk, two factors = medium risk and three or more factors = high risk. The higher the risk, the greater the intensity of monitoring required. It might be preferable not to prescribe opioids in high-risk patients or to refer them to a pain specialist.

Do not prescribe opioids if the patient has a condition for which opioids are not recommended (Table 3.4). A pain management programme and/or referral to a pain specialist are recommended.

Initiation of opioids

- Discuss advantages and disadvantages of opioid treatment with the patient, including short- and long-term side effects (Tables 3.7 and 3.8), tolerance, dependency and addiction.

- Record a pain score (from 0 to 10) using a visual analogue scale.

Short-term side effects of opioids

- Drowsiness
- Constipation
- Nausea and vomiting
- Urine retention
- Itching
- Respiratory depression

Table 3.7

Long-term side effects of opioids

- Suppression of the immune system
- Suppression of the hypothalamo–pituitary–adrenal axis, leading to hypogonadism, loss of libido, amenorrhoea, impaired fertility, possible suppression of adrenal function, low muscle mass, low bone mass, fatigue, depression and weight gain
- Impairment of cognitive function, especially memory and concentration
- Sweating
- Dry mouth
- Opioid-induced bowel disorder

Table 3.8

- If possible, use a quality-of-life scale (eg, the Brief Pain Inventory [BPI] or DoloTest) as a baseline and to monitor progress.

- In consultation with the patient, set three patient-specific goals (record these in the notes) – for example:

  - "What three things would you like to achieve by taking these drugs?"

  - Reduction in pain score (50–70% is the gold standard).

  - Improved sleep score (measured on the BPI).

- Functional goals – for example, being able to walk to the shops, play with children or swim three lengths of the pool.

- Explain the concept of an opioid trial and that the opioid will be tapered and stopped if the agreed goals are not achieved within the trial period of 6 weeks.

A supplementary video is available in the ebook version or from the Pain Community Centre website.

Opioids, immune and endocrine function | Joan Hester

▶ http://www.paincommunitycentre.org/article/opioids-immune-and-endocrine-function

Time required: 30 minutes

Opioid trial

- Plan for a 6-week trial.

- Use codeine or dihydrocodeine, if not used previously.

- Tramadol can be trialled, but remember that it is classed as a strong opioid (400 mg/day of tramadol is approximately equivalent to between 40 and 80 mg/day of oral morphine).

- If an alternative opioid is needed and there is no contraindication, use morphine, in either slow-release form (10–20 mg orally every 12 h) or immediate-release form (Oramorph® or Sevredol®; 5–10 mg every 4 h), as necessary to a maximum of 40 mg/day.

- If a lower dose is required, consider a 5–10 mcg/h buprenorphine skin patch for 7 days (10 mcg/h is approximately equivalent to 20 mg/day of oral morphine).

- If alternative opioids are required (eg, in patients with renal and liver impairment or sensitivity to morphine), check the morphine equivalence in the palliative care section of the *BNF* or local guidelines (eg, 25 mcg/h of transdermal fentanyl is equivalent to approximately 90 mg/day of oral morphine).

- Increase the dose every 2 weeks to a maximum of 120 mg of morphine, or equivalent, in 24 h. (In chronic non-malignant pain, for a total daily dose of above 120 mg of morphine, or equivalent, effectiveness might not increase and harm outweighs benefit.)

- Review the patient every 2 weeks, assess effectiveness and record side effects.
- At 6 weeks, assess the patient-specific goals, particularly functional goals, pain scores and side effects.
- If goals are achieved and there are acceptable or no side effects, proceed as follows:

    - Continue opioids.

    - Monitor the dose, pain score, function and side effects every 3 months.

    - Minimize 'top ups' and keep the daily dose as low as possible.

    - Monitor body-mass index (BMI) and blood pressure (use of opioids leads to weight gain and hypertension).

    - Monitor bone density (studies do not, as yet, give recommended time intervals).

    - Measure hormones (testosterone in men; luteinizing hormone, follicle-stimulating hormone and oestradiol in women) every 6 months and dehydroepiandrosterone (DHEAS) and early morning cortisol after 1 year.

    - If higher doses than 120 mg/day of morphine, or equivalent, are necessary, refer the patient to a specialist.

Reduction

If goals are not achieved and/or there are unacceptable side effects, proceed as follows:

- Taper opioids by 10–20 mg/day of morphine every 2 weeks until stopped completely.
- Consider switching to an alternative opioid if there are side effects – this is unlikely to improve effectiveness, however.
- Refer the patient to a specialist for further advice.

Important characteristics of individual opioids

This is not an inclusive list but a simple guide to features of practical concern; for further information, please consult local prescribing information or the *BNF:*

Codeine

- Metabolised to morphine in the liver.

- 10% of the population cannot convert codeine to morphine, so it might be ineffective. There are genetic and racial differences in the extent of hepatic metabolism.

- 240 mg/day of codeine (8 x 30 mg/day of strong Co-codamol®) is the equivalent of 30 mg/day of morphine.

- Constipating.

- Can cause epigastric pain or discomfort.

Dihydrocodeine

- A more potent form of codeine, but metabolic pathways are the same.

- 240 mg/day of dihydrocodeine is equivalent to 40 mg/day of morphine.

Tramadol

- Classified as a strong opioid in the *BNF*.

- Has to be metabolised to O-methyltramadol before it activates the mu receptor – onset of action is slow.

- Has a dual action – also acts as a weak inhibitor of the reuptake of serotonin and noradrenaline in the central nervous system, which might be the principal mode of action in some people.

- Wide individual variation in response.

- Withdrawal effects are common, even after a short period of dosing.

- Side effects are common, including sickness and headache.

Morphine

- Pharmacological effects are well-described – use as the 'standard' opioid, unless contraindicated.

- Has active metabolites, especially morphine-6-glucoronide (M-6-G), which is long-acting and excreted by the kidney – might accumulate in renal failure and lead to toxicity.

- Absorption via the oral route is variable (10–80%).

- Many different preparations are available – slow-release forms are commonly used.

- Short-term side effects occur in 80% of recipients but are usually manageable – for example early use of laxatives for constipation.

- Long-term adverse effects (endocrine system, immune system and cognitive function) are less well-understood but are important in long-term use.

- True allergy is rare but, if present, excludes admission to the Her Majesty's Armed Forces – causes histamine release, which can lead to a rash.

Oxycodone

- Twice as potent as morphine if given orally.

- Oral bioavailability is 60–80% – its absorption is more predictable compared with morphine.

- No active metabolites – it is metabolised by the cytochrome 450 (CYP) system in the liver, which is susceptible to genetic variation (p. 43).

- Caution is required in severe liver disease.

- High dependency and addiction potential.

- Potency is poorly recognised.

Fentanyl

- A highly potent opioid that can only be given transdermally (as a skin patch), via the oral mucosa (a sublingual tablet or lollipop) or by injection.

- Doses are in microgrammes, which can lead to confusion, so take great care when prescribing.

- A 25 mcg/h fentanyl skin patch is equivalent to approximately 90 mg/day of oral morphine (therefore, a 50 mcg/h fentanyl skin patch will be severely over the suggested upper limit of the recommended total daily dose of oral morphine [120 mg/day] in chronic non-malignant pain).

- Slow onset of action and continued effect for 18 h after application or removal of a skin patch.
- Short-acting forms are highly addictive and their use should be restricted to acute and cancer pain only.
- Side effects are the same as for other opioids, but it is perhaps less constipating.
- Opioid of choice in renal impairment.
- Dependency and withdrawal effects are common.
- Some patients might not remove previous patches, leading to toxicity from accumulating numbers of patches stuck onto the skin.
- External heat increases the rate of absorption and can lead to toxicity.
- Sweating is a common side effect.

Buprenorphine

- A partial agonist of the mu receptor.
- Does not antagonize the effect of morphine and other opioids in clinical practice.
- Most side effects are similar to those of other opioids.
- Lack of endocrine effects.
- Available as sublingual tablets and both low-strength (7-day) and higher-strength (3-day) skin patches – BuTrans® 5 mcg/h is equivalent to 10 mg/day of morphine or approximately 90 mg/day of codeine.
- Useful in liver disease and pancreatitis.
- Reputed to have a 'ceiling effect' for analgesia and side effects, but this is not apparent in clinical practice.

Tapentadol

- Licensed for use in severe pain in 2011 in the UK and has been used in Germany and the US for approximately 5 years, so there is limited clinical experience compared with other opioids.

- Has a dual effect on mu receptors and noradrenaline pathways in the central nervous system and therefore requires a smaller morphine-equivalent dose to achieve the same effect as a traditional opioid.
- Potentially fewer side effects than other opioids.
- Potential role in the treatment of neuropathic pain.
- Potentially less dependency.
- Withdrawal effects can occur if switching from other opioids to tapentadol (seek specialist advice).

Injected opioids have no place in the management of chronic non-malignant pain, so use them only in the management of acute pain and terminal illness.

Do not use pethidine for persistent pain. It has a short half-life, provides unpredictable analgesia and is metabolised to norpethidine, which is neurotoxic, causing convulsions and possible death.

No response to analgesic treatment with codeine or tramadol?

- Consider CYP2D6.
- Codeine and tramadol are the most commonly prescribed analgesics for moderate-to-severe pain, often prescribed in a 'trial-and-error' approach with other analgesics and adjuvants.
- Codeine and tramadol are considered pro-drugs, requiring bioactivation by the CYP2D6 enzyme to their respective active metabolites for analgesic efficacy. Therefore, a lack of response to codeine or tramadol could be because of polymorphisms in the *CYP2D6* gene, reducing enzyme function and the ability to biotransform these drugs to their effective metabolites.
- The *CYP2D6* gene is part of family 2, sub-family D, polypeptide 6 of the *CYP450* gene super-family, which is a large and functionally diverse group of genes located primarily in the liver. This gene super-family has a central role in drug metabolism and detoxification, with the *CYP2D6* gene encoding the CYP2D6 enzyme, which metabolises approximately 30% of all marketed drugs.
- The *CYP2D6* gene is highly polymorphic and >100 alleles have been identified, with new variations validated regularly.

- *CYP2D6* gene polymorphisms affect enzyme production and function – there are four validated phenotypes of CYP2D6 function:

  - Ultra-rapid metaboliser – individuals have multiple fully functional copies of the *CYP2D6* gene, leading to increased enzyme production. These individuals will rapidly metabolise tramadol and codeine, potentially leading to adverse drug reactions. There are multiple case reports, particularly in paediatrics, in which codeine has caused fatal morphine toxicity because of the ultra-rapid metaboliser phenotype. In 2013, the US Food and Drug Administration (FDA) issued a boxed warning that the use of codeine is contraindicated in children after tonsillectomy.

  - Extensive metaboliser – individuals have normal CYP2D6 enzyme function, ranging from 50–100%, which results in a normal response to codeine and tramadol.

  - Intermediate metaboliser – CYP2D6 function is reduced by 75%, resulting in a sub-optimal response to codeine and tramadol. These individuals are also at risk of adverse drug reactions from agents, such as amitriptyline, which are reliant on the CYP2D6 enzyme for clearance of active metabolites.

  - Poor metaboliser – individuals have limited or no CYP2D6 function and therefore cannot bioactivate codeine or tramadol. Similar to intermediate metabolisers, these individuals are also at risk of adverse drug reactions from agents that are reliant on the CYP2D6 enzyme for clearance of active metabolites.

- There is also ethnic variability in the prevalence of CYP2D6 phenotypes – for example, up to 29% of Saudi Arabians and Ethiopians are ultra-rapid metaboliser phenotypes compared with 5% of Caucasians. The Caucasian population is affected mostly by reduced function or inactive polymorphisms of the *CYP2D6* gene, leading to the intermediate metaboliser (10–15%) and poor metaboliser (7–10%) phenotypes.

- The CYP2D6 enzyme can be inhibited by other drugs, including herbal supplements, but is not readily induced:

  - Polypharmacy of multiple CYP2D6 substrates and pro-drugs co-prescribed with CYP2D6 inhibitors, particularly selective serotonin reuptake inhibitors (SSRIs), can inhibit the CYP2D6 enzyme – for example, an extensive metaboliser with normal CYP2D6 function can be reduced to a poor metaboliser with no CYP2D6 function by concomitant use of a single strong CYP2D6 enzyme inhibitor, such as fluoxetine or paroxetine.

  - The magnitude of CYP2D6 inhibition for several drugs has been clinically confirmed by the US FDA and other organizations (p. 124).

  - Weak-to-moderate inhibitors can reduce CYP2D6 function by up to 50%, whereas strong inhibitors can reduce CYP2D6 function by up to 100%.

  - Inhibition of the CYP2D6 enzyme can also occur if multiple substrates are co-prescribed. In substrate inhibition, there is a progressive decrease in CYP2D6 function at high substrate concentrations.

- A lack of response to codeine or tramadol could therefore be because of either *CYP2D6* genetic polymorphisms, leading to a poor or intermediate metaboliser phenotype, or CYP2D6 inhibition by poly-pharmacy.

Role of the GP

- If a sub-optimal response to codeine or tramadol is reported, consider switching to an alternative analgesic that is not reliant on CYP2D6 metabolism for its analgesic effect or changing the inhibitive concomitant drug.

- Referral to a pain specialist is recommended for the following:

  - Detailed pain assessment.

  - Diagnostic difficulties.

  - If alternative pain management is required – for example a pain management programme or interventions such as epidural injection or spinal cord stimulation.

- Opioid-insensitive pain.
- Patients with previous mental health problems, dependency and addiction.
- Special needs – for example, pregnancy, children, adolescents, older people or those with learning difficulties.
- Patients who are opioid-sensitive and might benefit from higher doses.
- Difficulty tapering.

Management of chronic LBP and sciatica

Sanjeeva Gupta and Manohar Sharma

Keywords

- Red flags.
- Yellow flags.
- Nociceptive pain.
- Neuropathic pain.
- Discogenic pain.
- Facet joint pain.
- Sacroiliac joint pain.
- Waddell's signs.
- Pharmacotherapy.
- Physical therapy.
- Referral.

Objectives

- To ensure that patients presenting with LBP are screened and assessed using current evidence-based approaches, ruling out red flags.
- To ensure that psychosocial factors, if present, are addressed (p. 12).
- To ensure that a provisional diagnosis can be made on which to guide management.

- To encourage and support self-management.
- To facilitate evidence-based management that includes drug, non-drug and interventional approaches.
- To identify when to refer to secondary care (eg, intractable pain, poor outcome from initial management or diagnostic dilemma).

Background

- Non-specific mechanical LBP is common.
- LBP is one of the commonest reasons for sickness and loss of revenue.
- Most episodes of non-specific LBP settle with conservative management in the community.
- In a small number of patients, LBP becomes disabling and chronic.
- Biopsychosocial factors are crucial in managing chronic LBP because pain-related fear, catastrophizing, anxiety and mood, for example, can be barriers to recovery.
- In many cases, it can be difficult to find the cause of the pain with the usual biomedical model, for example history-taking, examination and various investigations.
- Structures that might cause LBP include, but are not limited to, the following:
  - Intervertebral discs.
  - Facet joints.
  - Sacroiliac joints.
  - Muscles.
  - Ligaments.
  - Vertebral body (collapse, fracture, spine instability or malignancy).
- LBP can be caused by the following pathologies:
  - Degenerative spine changes.
  - Inflammatory conditions.
  - Metabolic conditions.

- Infection.
- Metastatic deposits.
- Multiple myeloma.
- LBP can be caused by pathology in other parts of body, for example:
  - Pelvic – ovarian or uterine pathologies.
  - Abdominal – for example, aortic aneurysm, kidney-related pathologies, chronic pancreatitis or secondary tumours involving para-aortic lymph nodes.
- LBP can be associated with radicular pain in the lower limbs, resulting from disc prolapse, or foramenal stenosis, causing nerve root or spinal cord compression.

Assessment

History-taking

- Age and gender of the patient.
- How did the LBP start?
- History of trauma or road traffic accident?
- Aggravating and relieving factors.
- Character of pain – nociceptive and/or neuropathic pain.
- Family history of LBP and inflammatory conditions.
- Family history of infective diseases like tuberculosis.
- Previous and current treatment for LBP.
- History of co-morbidities, for example respiratory, cardiac, central nervous system, gastrointestinal, renal or hepatic conditions, which can influence the choice of pharmacotherapy.
- Drug allergies.

Examination

- Neurological examination.
- Rule out red flags (Table 3.9).
- Any neurological signs to confirm radicular/neuropathic pain?

Red flags: signs or symptoms that need further investigation or referral

History

- Previous history of malignancy
- Age <16 or >50 years with new-onset pain
- Weight loss (unexplained)
- Previous longstanding steroid use
- Recent serious illness
- Recent significant infection
- Recent significant trauma

Symptoms

- Non-mechanical pain (worse at rest)
- Thoracic pain
- Fevers/rigors
- General malaise
- Urinary retention
- Faecal incontinence

Signs

- Saddle anaesthesia
- Loss of anal tone
- Multilevel sensory-motor deficits

Table 3.9

- Midline pain in younger patients that is worse on flexion could be discogenic pain.
- Paraspinal pain that is worse on lumbar spine extension and rotation could originate in the facet joint.
- LBP in a multiparous female patient, which is most severe below the fifth lumbar vertebra (L5 spinal level) is more likely to be mediated by the sacroiliac joint.
- Look for Waddell's Signs (Table 3.10) – the behavioural response to examination should be interpreted carefully.

Multiple positive signs could suggest that the patient might not have a simple physical problem and so consider psychological factors. The patient might require management of psychological and behavioural problems, in addition to the physical pathology, if present.

Diagnosis

- Non-specific LBP.

- Although difficult to diagnose by the history and examination, consider the specific causes of LBP:

  - Discogenic low back pain.

Waddell's signs
Tenderness tests
• Superficial tenderness to light touch on the skin
• Non-anatomical tenderness – the pattern of tenderness does relate to the anatomical structure
Simulation tests
• Gentle pressure on the top of the head produces a complaint of back pain
• Rotation – reproduction of back pain if the pelvis and shoulder are passively rotated in the same plane when the patient stands with feet together and is relaxed
Distraction tests
• A positive physical finding is checked while the patient is distracted. A patient whose back pain has a non-organic component shows marked improvement in straight-leg raising on distraction compared with formal testing
Regional disturbances
• Sudden or uneven weakness on strength-testing ('give-way weakness')
• Non-anatomical sensory changes
Over-reaction
• Exaggerated responses or responses that cannot be reproduced

Table 3.10

- Facet joint-mediated pain.
- Sacroiliac joint pain.
- Spinal stenosis.
- Predominant radicular pain – sciatica.
- Inflammatory conditions – rheumatoid arthritis and ankylosing spondylitis.

Screening

- Blood tests for inflammatory markers.
- The role of x-ray is limited, unless there is a history of trauma.
- A computed tomography (CT) scan is helpful if bone-related causes are suspected.
- The role of ultrasound is limited, unless to rule out other abdominal causes of LBP.
- A magnetic resonance imaging (MRI) scan has high sensitivity but low specificity to help with the diagnosis.
- An MRI scan should only be considered if red flags are suspected and injection therapy or surgery is planned to define the target level for the intervention.

Good clinical practice

- If red flags are present, refer the patient immediately to specialized services.
- Identify yellow flags and address them in the community.
- Identify the possible source of LBP.
- Identify whether the patient has radicular pain, because treatment is different.
- Treat pain aggressively to prevent chronicity – with frequent follow-up to review progress.
- Refer early for physical therapy to encourage and support self-management.
- Explain the cause of pain and its management to the patient – shared decision-making helps to develop a management plan that both patient and clinician support.

- If LBP does not settle, reassess using the STarT back tool to guide further management.

Management

- Treat persistent LBP and radicular pain according to the British Pain Society and Map of Medicine LBP and radicular pain pathway/guidelines and up-to-date evidence-based guidelines.
- Advice/self-management.
- Acute LBP does get better on its own quite quickly, mostly within 6 weeks.
- Stress can increase the pain felt and tension can cause muscle spasm – encourage relaxation and simple, relaxed breathing.
- Do not be frightened by the pain, hurt does not mean harm.
- Encourage the patient to remain as active as the pain allows, checking that posture is good. Taking rest periods before the pain gets worse is also helpful (pacing).
- Regular exercises, as advised by a physical therapist, will help quicker recovery.
- There is good evidence that keeping active speeds up recovery. Bed rest for more than 1–2 days is neither beneficial nor recommended.
- There will be flare-ups during the recovery period and this is normal.
- Regular analgesics, including anti-inflammatories (if appropriate), will enable activity and speed recovery.

Pharmacotherapy

- Non-specific LBP is multimodal analgesia, using analgesics that act by different mechanisms and at different sites along the pain pathway provide optimal analgesia with least side effects. Consider neuropathic pain and if present treat it early. If nociceptive LBP and neuropathic lower limb pain are present, both will need treating:
  - Paracetamol.
  - NSAIDs, if there are no contraindications.

- Weak opioids.
- Avoid strong opioids.
- Treat neuropathic pain with TCAs, gabapentenoids and sodium-channel blockers – multimodal analgesia might be necessary in some patients.
- Management of side effects associated with drug management.
- In the acute phase, regular use of analgesics is more likely to help compared with use 'as needed'.

Non-drug management, including return to work

- Advise on the usefulness of physical therapy and agree a management plan using appropriate and evidence-based approaches:
  - Physiotherapy.
  - Manipulative therapy.
  - Acupuncture.
  - TENS.
- Assess the need for pain relief to support physical therapy.
- Encourage and build pacing and coping, and lifting and handling techniques.
- Refer the patient to occupational therapy for advice about returning to work.
- The individual might need to return to work in a phased manner.

Management plan, including referral pathways and technological approaches

- Refer the patient to a specialist centre if the pain is not improving or the patient has radicular pain not improving with pharmacotherapy (p. 121). Management in specialist centres might include the following:
  - Non-drug treatments, including physiotherapy and a trial of TENS.

- Pharmacological management with TCAs, gabapentenoids and sodium-channel blockers for neuropathic pain.

- Diagnostic medial branch block followed by radiofrequency denervation for LBP from the facet joints.

- Image-guided (fluoroscopy) early epidural steroid injections and transforaminal epidurals for LBP with radicular pain.

- Nucleoplasty could be indicated if the disc is contained within the annulus fibrosis and image-guided epidural steroid injections have not helped.

- Injection of local anaesthetic and steroid into the sacroiliac joint can be diagnostic as well as therapeutic. Radiofrequency denervation of the sacroiliac joint could be considered if the pain relief from the sacroiliac joints is short-lived.

- Referral to a surgical team is indicated if epidural steroid injections have not helped and the disc is extruded.

- Patients with persistent LBP can benefit from referral to the pain management programme (cognitive-behavioural-therapy-based pain management programme).

Role of the GP

- Assess and screen the patient, ensuring that red flags are ruled out and any psychosocial factors of note are incorporated into the management plan.

- Reassure and educate patients who present with acute LBP because often the pain is likely to settle with conservative management; advise about posture, lifting and handling, pacing and coping, and regular physiotherapy exercise.

- Identify self-management support and encourage the patient to consider adopting principles early on.

- Refer early for physical therapy.

- Advise on healthy living and smoking cessation, because the evidence suggests poor outcomes and recovery in smokers.

- Manage pain aggressively:
  - Multimodal analgesia.
  - Consider neuropathic pain and, if present, treat appropriately.

- Encourage gradual return to normal activity with good analgesia.

- Avoid strong opioids.

- If pain is not getting better, reassess within 2 weeks of the initial presentation using the STarT Back tool to guide further management.

- Refer to a specialist centre if the pain is not responding to primary care management.

Chronic widespread pain and fibromyalgia

Benjamin Ellis

Keywords

- Risk factors.
- Musculoskeletal.
- Fibromyalgia.
- Pharmacological management.
- Psychological management.

Objectives

- To identify the risk factors for chronic widespread pain and fibromyalgia.

- To discuss assessment, screening and diagnosis of chronic widespread pain and fibromyalgia.

- To present the evidence-based treatment options and self-management approaches.

Background

- Chronic widespread pain can be defined as pain lasting more than 3 months and affecting both sides of the body, as well as sites above and below the waist, plus pain in the axial skeleton.

- Around 1 in 10 people in the UK general population are affected, which is similar to estimates in other countries.

- In common with other musculoskeletal pain syndromes, prevalence has markedly increased over the last 50 years.

- On reading the following, it will become apparent, as with other complex pain conditions, that the primary care practitioner is unlikely to achieve all that is required in a standard 10-minute consultation. Therefore, it is anticipated that multiple assessments will be needed over several months, with the same health professional.

Risk factors

- Individual risk factors for chronic widespread pain include female sex, rising age, obesity, and poor mental and physical health, in addition to prior life stress and physical trauma in the months before onset.

- A positive family history is commonly seen, because fibromyalgia tends to aggregate in families.

- Persistent health-seeking behaviour, somatization and poor sleep are independently predictive of an increased risk of developing chronic widespread pain.

- Persistence is seen in half of people at 1 year and one-third of people at 7 years.

- As well as an adverse impact on quality of life and social and work participation, chronic widespread pain has been associated with a significant increase in mortality.

Relationships between pain syndromes

- Chronic widespread pain is generally considered to be a continuum of symptoms, with fibromyalgia the most severe clinical manifestation. Around one-fifth of people with chronic widespread pain meet the classic American College of Rheumatology 1990 criteria for fibromyalgia, which require the presence of tender points on clinical examination.

- Transition to chronic widespread pain occurs in around one in five of those with chronic regional pain syndromes such as back pain.

- Neuroimaging techniques have shown changes in neuroreceptor binding patterns, anatomical structure and metabolite activity in the brains of people with fibromyalgia, implicating abnormal central pain processing as a likely aetiology. Twin studies have suggested genetic susceptibility, but no genes have yet been definitively identified.

Benefits of making a diagnosis

Patients with chronic widespread pain or fibromyalgia should be given their diagnosis. Receiving a diagnostic label of fibromyalgia does not worsen long-term health outcome and, on the contrary, by enabling an appropriate therapeutic approach, might reduce both number and severity of symptoms and increase satisfaction with health. Similarly, in the initial years after a diagnosis of fibromyalgia is received, there is a reduction in the patient's use of health services, although this is not maintained in the long term. Unfortunately, it is acknowledged that some healthcare practitioners 'do not believe' in the existence of fibromyalgia. Belief and empathy are important facets of treatment.

Assessment

Who should be assessed?

- Many patients with chronic widespread pain will already be known to the clinician.

- Before diagnosis, many patients will have been seen repeatedly for other painful conditions, including regional pain syndromes, chest pain and headache, as well as non-painful problems such as depression, fatigue, sleep disturbance, irritable bowel syndrome and dizziness.

- Recurrent presentations with these disorders should trigger further enquiry about widespread pain (Figure 3.2).

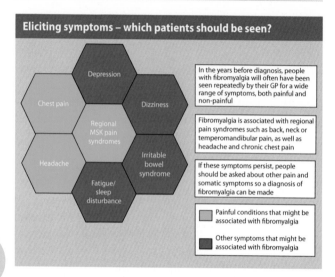

Eliciting symptoms – which patients should be seen?

Depression

Chest pain

Dizziness

Regional MSK pain syndromes

Headache

Irritable bowel syndrome

Fatigue/ sleep disturbance

In the years before diagnosis, people with fibromyalgia will often have been seen repeatedly by their GP for a wide range of symptoms, both painful and non-painful

Fibromyalgia is associated with regional pain syndromes such as back, neck or temperomandibular pain, as well as headache and chronic chest pain

If these symptoms persist, people should be asked about other pain and somatic symptoms so a diagnosis of fibromyalgia can be made

Painful conditions that might be associated with fibromyalgia

Other symptoms that might be associated with fibromyalgia

Figure 3.2 GP, general practitioner; MSK, musculoskeletal. Courtesy of Benjamin Ellis.

What are the main symptoms to elicit?

- Assess the duration, extent, severity and nature of pain.

- Establish whether there is persistent pain in all four body quadrants, in addition to axial pain, lasting more than 3 months.

- Determine whether there are additional features present, in particular cognitive and somatic symptoms, as well as poor sleep and fatigue. These can be formally assessed to fulfil the 2010 American College of Rheumatology criteria for fibromyalgia, which allow a diagnosis to be made without physical examination.

- Somatic symptoms to explore include the presence of dry eyes/ mouth, peripheral paraesthesia and bladder/bowel pattern.

- Enquire about mood and consider completing a structured questionnaire such as PHQ-9.

- Undertake an assessment of the impact of pain and associated symptoms on the person's life, including family, intimate, social and work participation.

Perform a clinical examination of painful areas and to exclude other pathology

- Examine any focal painful areas, looking for evidence of abnormalities.

- Carry out a musculoskeletal system screening examination, for example the Gait, Arms, Legs and Spine (GALS) screen.

- A tender-point examination can be done to look for sensitivity to pressure, as described in the 1990 American College of Rheumatology criteria for fibromyalgia.

- Complete a neurological examination, looking for evidence of weakness or upper motor neurone signs.

- Palpate the neck, axillae and groin for lymphadenopathy.

- Note the presence of finger/toenail abnormalities, skin rashes, psoriasis, skin or mouth ulceration and alopecia.

- Examine any other systems identified in the history as abnormal.

Diagnostic investigations to check

- Collect a urine sample and dipstick test for the presence of blood, protein or glucose.

- Send blood tests for the following:

  - Full blood count (FBC).

  - Urea and electrolytes (U&Es).

  - Liver function tests (LFTs).

  - Bone profile.

  - Erythrocyte sedimentation rate (ESR).

  - Thyroid function tests (TFTs).

  - Fasting glucose.

- The following tests are not routinely indicated:

  - Rheumatoid factor (RF).

  - Anti-nuclear antibody (ANA).

  - Anti-neutrophil cytoplasmic antibody (ANCA).

  - Immunoglobulins (Igs).

  - Creatine kinase (CK).

- If inflammatory arthritis is suspected on the basis of stiffness, swelling or metacarpophalangeal (MCP)/ metatarsophalangeal (MTP) joint tenderness, the patient needs urgent referral to specialist rheumatology services and there is no added benefit to checking rheumatoid serology.

- Vitamin D levels – clear evidence linking chronic widespread pain in the general population to hypovitaminosis D is lacking and routine checking of baseline vitamin D levels is not indicated unless there are abnormalities of bone profile, additional physical signs or the patient is in a high-risk group for developing the condition.

Review of risk factors for poor outcome

- Consider early referral to specialist multidisciplinary pain services for assessment and treatment for people with poor prognostic factors, as well as those who do not improve with initial primary care-based treatment.

- Risk factors for persistence include age over 50 years, daytime tiredness, and dry eyes and mouth, as well as severity and extent of pain, poor functional and mental capacity, and levels of psychological distress.

- People with high levels of depression are likely to have poorer outcomes in pain, physical functioning and quality of life after receiving multidisciplinary treatment for their fibromyalgia.

- Alcohol misuse should be considered a marker for poor psychological health, increasing the risk of poor outcomes.

- Significant physical health co-morbidities might have an adverse effect on outcome.

- The use of 'yellow, blue and black flags' provides a framework for identifying factors likely to lead to poor outcomes (Figure 3.3).

Red flags

- The presence of the following symptoms should raise the possibility of other pathology. If present, consider referral to specialist care for investigation:

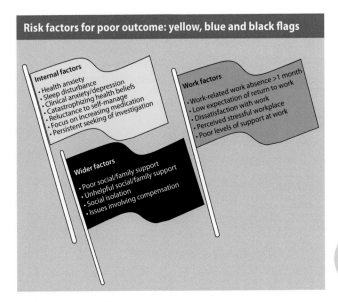

Risk factors for poor outcome: yellow, blue and black flags

Internal factors
- Health anxiety
- Sleep disturbance
- Clinical anxiety/depression
- Catastrophizing health beliefs
- Reluctance to self-manage
- Focus on increasing medication
- Persistent seeking of investigation

Work factors
- Work-related work absence >1 month
- Low expectation of return to work
- Dissatisfaction with work
- Perceived stressful workplace
- Poor levels of support at work

Wider factors
- Poor social/family support
- Unhelpful social/family support
- Social isolation
- Issues involving compensation

Figure 3.3 Courtesy of Benjamin Ellis.

- Early morning stiffness in joints (lasting over 30 minutes), focal joint pain or swelling.

- Weight loss or fever.

- Raynaud's phenomenon of recent origin.

- Dry eyes/mouth.

- Skin rashes or ulcers, or alopecia.

- Personal or family history of inflammatory arthritis, psoriasis or inflammatory bowel disease.

- Visual change, or red or painful eyes.

- Sensory changes, muscle weakness or cramp.

- Lymphadenopathy.

- Abnormal neurological signs present (including muscle abnormalities).

- Swollen joints (synovitis), or MCP or MTP joint tenderness/ pain on squeeze test (urgent referral).

- Unexplained blood/protein on urine dipstick.
- Unexplained rise in ESR.

Patient education

- Provide information about chronic widespread pain or fibromyalgia (Figure 3.4):

  - Outline the nature of the disorder as an abnormality of central pain processing.

  - Offer printed disorder-specific information (available from a range of organizations; p. 63).

  - Emphasise that although there is no 'cure', most people can substantially improve their symptoms and quality of life by engaging in a treatment programme.

  - Clarify that treatment involves multiple approaches, of which medication is only one.

  - Promote the benefits of remaining physically active and engaged in normal activities at a sustainable level, including working as relevant.

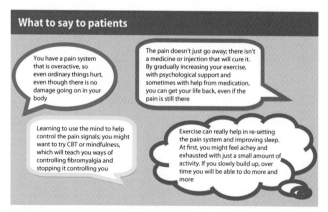

What to say to patients

You have a pain system that is overactive, so even ordinary things hurt, even though there is no damage going on in your body

The pain doesn't just go away; there isn't a medicine or injection that will cure it. By gradually increasing your exercise, with psychological support and sometimes with help from medication, you can get your life back, even if the pain is still there

Learning to use the mind to help control the pain signals; you might want to try CBT or mindfulness, which will teach you ways of controlling fibromyalgia and stopping it controlling you

Exercise can really help in re-setting the pain system and improving sleep. At first, you might feel achey and exhausted with just a small amount of activity. If you slowly build up, over time you will be able to do more and more

Figure 3.4 CBT, cognitive-behavioural therapy. Courtesy of Benjamin Ellis and Tom Margham.

- Suggest simple self-management approaches, such as bathing and stretching in warm water.
- Encourage self-management, including giving people a copy of *The Pain Toolkit* (p. 118) and/or the details of the website (http://www.paintoolkit.org/).

Signpost to other sources of support:

- Direct people toward organizations that provide information and/or support for people with chronic widespread pain or fibromyalgia, for example:
  - Action on Pain.
  - Arthritis Care.
  - Arthritis Research UK.
  - Fibromyalgia UK (FMA UK).
  - Pain Concern.
- Suggest participation in structured self-management programmes, including the following:
  - Expert patient programme, including online courses.
  - Arthritis Care 'Challenging Pain' course.
  - Help identify sources of peer support.
  - Give information about benefits, if appropriate.
  - Suggest social services, if support services are needed.
  - Citizens advice centres for a range of options.
  - Personal independence services (eg, for equipment).

Drug management

General guidance on drug management for patients with chronic non-malignant pain is provided on p. 28.

General principles of medication therapy for chronic widespread pain

- Agree goals of therapy before prescribing and adjust the choice of medications to meet the needs of the individual.

- Discuss risks and benefits of potential medications, in particular discuss potential side effects.

- Explore alternatives to pharmacological therapies for pain management.

- It is important to recognise that only up to 50% of people with fibromyalgia derive some benefit from medication.

- Give medication an adequate therapeutic trial and agree this period with the patient at treatment initiation – some medications might require dose titration and optimization over several weeks before reaching maximum therapeutic effect.

- Consider scheduling a planned review 2–4 weeks after each medication change.

- At planned medication reviews, use the four 'A's as a framework (p. 32):

  - Analgesia – is the medication still providing useful pain relief?

  - Adverse effects – what side effects is the patient experiencing and can these be managed more effectively?

  - Activity – does the patient maintain suitable physical and psychosocial functioning?

  - Adherence – is the patient taking medication as agreed in the management plan?

Specific drug treatments for use in chronic widespread pain and fibromyalgia

- Evidence for drug efficacy comes from studies in fibromyalgia (Table 3.11).

- Explain that effective treatments are generally central nervous system agents working to modulate pain pathways involving neurotransmitters, such as noradrenaline or serotonin, although the drugs were developed for other purposes such as to treat epilepsy or depression.

- Explain that treatments must be taken regularly to be effective, usually for several weeks.

Primary care medication management for fibromyalgia

Drug	Comments	Dosage
Tricyclic antidepressants	These drugs have good evidence for efficacy	
Amitriptyline	Take in the mid-evening; can improve sleep and pain	Initally 10 mg/day; titrate up, as appropriate
Nortriptyline	Similar to amitriptyline; might have fewer side effects	Initially 10 mg/day; titrate up, as appropriate
Anticonvulsants	These drugs can improve pain, sleep and overall quality of life	
Gabapentin		Initially 300 mg once daily; titrate up to 1200–2400 mg/day
Pregabalin		Initially 150 mg/day; titrate up to 450 mg/day
Tramadol	Unlike opioids, tramadol is often of benefit in fibromyalgia, probably because of induction of serotonin release and inhibition of noradrenaline reuptake	50–100 mg four times daily
SSRIs	Demonstrate benefit over placebo	
Fluoxetine		20–80 mg/day
SNRIs	Dual uptake inhibitors can also be effective	
Duloxetine		60 mg twice daily
Vitamin D	In some population subsets (or if vitamin D deficiency is specifically suspected), a trial of oral vitamin D therapy should be considered	800 units daily (or follow local protocol)

Table 3.11 SNRI, serotonin–norepinephrine reuptake inhibitor; SSRI, selective serotonin reuptake inhibitor.

Non-drug management, including return to work

- There is good evidence of efficacy for a wide range of approaches rooted in supported self-management, physical therapies and psychological support.

- Cognitive-behavioural therapies improve pain, fatigue, mood and function in fibromyalgia, and the benefits can last many months – consider referral for other psychological interventions, including meditation, relaxation and stress management, all of which have demonstrated benefit in fibromyalgia.

- Physical activity, both cardiovascular exercise and strength training, reduces pain for people with fibromyalgia, and *T'ai Chi* seems to be of benefit – consider referral to physiotherapy, ideally delivered by pain-specialist physiotherapists, for graded exercise programmes.

- Educational interventions, including structured education programmes focussing on self-management, can produce a sustained improvement in symptoms.

- Refer to a sleep clinic or insomnia services – sleep disturbance is a major symptom reducing quality of life, and improved sleep has been linked to resolution of chronic widespread pain (p. 105).

- Consider referral to occupational therapy or occupational health services for rehabilitation for social and work participation.

- Ideally, all these interventions should be delivered as an integrated programme of physical activity with a range of psychosocial interventions. This might be possible through referral to a pain management programme.

- Cognitive-behavioural therapy might be helpful for managing pain and fatigue, and their impact, as well as pain-related fear and treating anxiety/depression – consider online cognitive-behavioural therapy as an alternative option for some people.

Side-effect management

- As with any medical treatment, some people might experience side effects, and common and serious side effects should be discussed with patients before starting a new treatment.

- It is possible that sensory processing abnormalities in widespread persistent pain and fibromyalgia might increase the number and severity of bothersome side effects.

- Discuss with patients that some side effects will reduce in severity over time, and therefore they might wish to persevere with a medication to see whether they will benefit.

- Morning drowsiness is a common side effect of amitriptyline taken the night before and might be helped by taking the medication earlier in the evening.

Management plan, including referral pathways and technological approaches

- Referral to specialist care for diagnosis might be required if red flags or other features suggestive of an alternative diagnosis are present.

- Referral to specialist care for treatment might be required if either there are features suggestive of a poor prognosis from the outset or people do not benefit from a trial of optimal primary care-based treatment.

- Referrals to community specialist allied health professionals in psychology, physiotherapy, occupational therapy and others might be required (p. 66).

Role of the GP

- Believe and support the patient.
- Perform adequate and ongoing assessment of the condition.
- Initiate, titrate, monitor and stop appropriate medication.
- Support ongoing self-management.
- Make appropriate referrals.

Pelvic pain

John Hughes

Keywords

- Chronic pelvic pain syndrome (CPPS).
- Cyclical pain.

Objectives

- To assess the patient as a whole (biological, psychological and social aspects), including undertaking a history, examination and any investigations.

- To consider and manage known defined conditions accordingly (eg, urinary tract infection, acute pyelonephritis or suspected cancer).

- To consider concurrent managing as CPPS, if symptoms persist with a well-defined condition that is being adequately managed.

- To improve patients' understanding of pelvic pain and direct patients to recourses for pelvic pain specifically.

- To consider combinations of agents aimed at differing elements of the condition.

- To form a management plan to improve function (quality of life), which must be agreed by the patient and clinician.

- To provide the patient with the skills to manage their own pain.

- To understand when to refer to specialist services if progress is not achieved in a reasonable time (6 months from presentation).

Background

- Chronic pelvic pain is chronic or persistent pain perceived in structures related to the pelvis of either men or women.

- It is often associated with negative cognitive, behavioural, sexual and emotional consequences, as well as with symptoms suggestive of lower urinary tract and sexual, bowel, pelvic floor or gynaecological dysfunction. Patients must be taken seriously and assessed, even if the history does not fit with the known symptom patterns for common conditions.

- In the case of documented nociceptive pain that becomes chronic/persistent over time, pain must have been continuous or recurrent for at least 6 months – that is, it can be cyclical over a 6-month period, such as the cyclical pain of dysmenorrhoea.

- CPPS is the occurrence of chronic pelvic pain in the absence of proven infection or other obvious local pathology that might account for the pain.

- Pelvic pain is common, affecting an estimated one million women in the UK.

- It assumes that well-defined pelvic pathologies have been excluded and managed accordingly.

- Manage conditions with known pathologies that present as pelvic pain accordingly (specific pathways might already exist). This could include referral to the appropriate specialist.

- If there are sudden changes in presentation, consider the possibility of new pathology or an acute cause.

- Only consider repeat investigations if the clinical picture suggests they might be beneficial in planning future management.

- Allow sufficient time taking the history and undertaking an examination, as appropriate.

Assessment

- General history of the presenting complaint, including bowel, bladder and menstrual changes (if appropriate).

- History of the pain from onset to the present, including severity, exacerbating and easing factors, and radiation and its nature.

- Previous and present treatments.

- Include assessment of the effects on daily living.

- Review mood, sleep, anxiety, depression and unrewarding sexual encounters.

- Examine the localized area of pain, in addition to posture, range of movement, muscle function and tenderness. Include those local to the area of pain and those in the common referral projections. Consider internal examinations.

Pathway

It is important to have a logical approach to assessing and examining the patient with pelvic pain (Table 3.12).

Red flags

These are presentations or changes in presentation that should be considered and might require further investigation or referral to exclude treatable conditions (Table 3.13).

They might be present at the initial assessment or become apparent at follow-up – always take red flags seriously.

Diagnosis

- If a well-defined condition exists, treat and manage accordingly. Specific pathways might already exist for management or referral to the appropriate specialty (eg, prostatism, inflammatory bowel disease and dysmenorrhoea).
- CPPS is not a single entity and might be localized and perceived in the area of a single organ (eg, bladder or prostate) or more widespread. The aim is, therefore, to develop a management plan rather than make a specific diagnosis.
- Consider well-defined conditions that are optimally treated but continue to be painful for concurrent management as CPPS.

Good clinical practice

In managing the patient with pelvic pain, Table 3.14 presents some thoughts on good clinical practice.

Management

Develop a management plan with the patient and include ongoing assessment:

- Likely to be multifaceted, with biological, psychological and social elements.
- Include elements of self-management and goal-setting.
- Goal-setting should be realistic and involve the patient.

Assessment pathway

Structure of assessment

- Allow the patient to use their own words to describe their pain
- Use open questions to facilitate patients using their own words
- Use sensitive non-judgemental questioning, especially if broaching sensitive areas of sexual function and unrewarding sexual encounters
- Closed questions might help clarify details (eg, effect of bladder emptying)
- Summarize understanding back to the patient to clarify the presentation

What to ask

Pain	• Onset, development over time with localization and radiation. Cause, if known
	• Easing and exacerbating features, in addition to severity and variations
Bladder	• Frequency day and night
	• Urge and urgency
	• Pain related to bladder filling and emptying
	• Hesitancy, dysfunctional flow and incontinence
Bowel	• Frequency, consistency and straining
	• Urge and urgency, in addition to incontinence
	• Pain related to bowel function before, during and after defaecation
Menstrual cycle	• Relation of pain to the menstrual cycle
	• Dysmenorrhoea and menorrhagia
	• Altered cycle pattern
Effect on daily life	• Sleep, mood, anxiety and depression
	• Walking, sitting and standing
	• Concentration and fatigue

Table 3.12 CT, computed tomography; MRI, magnetic resonance imaging; STD, sexually transmitted disease; U/S, ultrasound; UTI, urinary tract infection.

- Desire to socialize or pursue hobbies
- Relations with others (social, family and work)
- Sexual functioning, including unrewarding sexual encounters both current and historical
- Include ability to perform, in addition to avoidance
- Severity of effect (eg, mild, moderate or severe)

Past medical history

- Review past history (eg, UTIs, STDs or congenital anomalies)

Patient perceptions

- What does the patient fear might be the problem?
- Anxieties about, for example, cancer, employability or fertility

Examination

- Allow time for the examination to be undertaken in a compassionate manner. Further details of the history or anxieties might be elucidated
- Assess the area the patient localized for pain

Skin	· Changes, including infection and trauma
Sensation	· Light touch and pin-prick
Range of movement	· Posture, standing and sitting, both static and functional
	· Movements – lumber, pelvis and hips, both passive and active
Muscle function	· Localized to the area of pain and in the common referral patterns
	· Length, stiffness and tenderness, including trigger points
	· Assess perineum
Internal examination	· Per rectum, vaginal or both
	· Often helpful to exclude well-defined conditions and red flags
	· Include the ease of penetration, muscle tension, tenderness, localization and muscle function

Table 3.12 Continued.

Investigations	
	• Avoid repeating investigations, unless it helps diagnostically
	• Repeated investigations might have a negative impact on patients' expectations of management
Simple tests	• Swabs and cultures (eg, midstream urine and *Chlamydia*)
Simple investigations	• U/S and MRI for known pathologies
	• Barium studies, CT or MRI, and endoscopy might be available but, if in doubt, speak to the appropriate speciality
Complex investigations	• Such as urodynamics and anorectal physiology – might require specialist referral

Table 3.12 Continued.

Red flags	
Gynaecology	Post-coital bleeding
	Pelvic mass
	Irregular vaginal bleeding over the age of 40 years
	New-onset postmenopausal pain
	Postmenopausal bleeding
Urological	Haematuria
	Urinary tract infection in men
Gastroenterological	Blood in stools
	Weight loss
	Night-time symptoms
	New bowel symptoms over the age of 50 years
	Family history of cancer or inflammatory bowel disease
	Anaemia
Psychological	Suicidal ideation with intent
	Major depressive disorder
	Other severe psychiatric illness

Table 3.13 This is not an exhaustive list.

> **Good clinical practice**
>
> - Be non-judgemental and allow the patient to use their own words
> - Use open questioning to allow the patient to explain their condition
> - Assess the impact on daily function (physical, emotional and environmental)
> - Involve the patient in the discussion – explore their anxieties and fears
> - Assess severity of effect (eg, mild, moderate or severe; 0 to 10 scale)
> - Assess the patient's expectations of outcome
> - Set realistic goals with the patient's active involvement
> - Record outcomes of interventions, including side effects of medications, doses and combinations used

Table 3.14

- High levels of fear and anxiety or major mood changes might benefit from a more psychological approach.

- Assess outcomes, including benefits, side effects, compliance and a general assessment of outcome.

- Pre-set a time for review.

Treatment targets

Treatment targets should be realistic and achievable across all aspects of daily functioning and quality of life. Undertake a balanced assessment, reviewing both positive and negative elements (Table 3.15).

Options

- The aim of management is to help the patient improve their daily functioning and overall quality of life.

- CPPS involves multiple mechanisms, both peripheral and central, and management requires a holistic approach.

- There are few medication studies specifically looking at CPPS, the evidence is therefore drawn from other neuropathic models of pain.

Treatment targets	
Physical	General daily activities
	Mobility, including walking and transferring
	Intimate relations
Psychology	Mood
	Sleep
	Anxiety
	Relationships (home, work and friends)
Medication	Balance of benefits
	Side effects
	Compliance
Expectations	Review the overall balance of change against goals
	Assess reasons for failure
	Set new goals with the patient

Table 3.15

- The focus of management will depend on the focus of presentation and patient preferences. It is likely to be multifaceted.

Patient education

- Patient involvement with their own care improves outcome.
- Patient understanding might reduce fear and aid self-management.
- Educating the patient enables them to be more active in their management plan.
- Recourses specific to pelvic pain or more general.

Drug management

- Multiple mechanisms are involved in CPPS and single agents might not have the optimal effect.

- Few studies look specifically at medications for CPPS, so the agents used are taken from the broader evidence base for central and neuropathic pain.
- Titrate doses in a planned fashion, with regular review to assess effect and compliance.

Options

- Simple analgesics for somatic pain (eg, cyclical pain).
- Co-analgesics for visceral or neuropathic pain, including TCAs, anticonvulsants and newer antidepressants.
- Use opioids with care and reference to the guidelines available.
- Consider the oral contraceptive for hormonally influenced pain.
- Consider agents affecting bladder or bowel function, if appropriate.

Side-effect management

- A balanced management plan incorporating the biopsychosocial model provides the best outcome.
- Compliance will influence outcome across all interventions.
- Patient understanding and involvement improves compliance.
- Understanding the patient's expectation of outcome is important if the best results are to be achieved.

Management plan

- Often patients can be optimally managed in primary care.
- Secondary care options might be a general pain management unit or a specialist urogenital unit.
- General and specialist units have access to a broader assessment, as well as more complex investigations and interventions.
- Specialist units have greater experience with complex cases and access to multidisciplinary working, which will include the primary care physician.

Management

- Review the management plan against outcome(s).
- If there is a significant benefit and side effects are tolerated, maintain the plan.
- If side effects outweigh benefit, review the plan.
- If no benefit persists, consider referral to specialist services.
- Regular agreed review of outcome.
- Review progress from the previous visit.
- Discharge back to self-care if the patient is stable and in agreement.
- Continue review, with an agreed timeline, if the patient is stable but not ready for self-care.
- Refer to specialist services if progress is slow or inadequate.

Role of the GP

- Assess for well-defined conditions and treat or refer accordingly.
- Involve the patient with the management plan.
- Review the response to interventions.
- Refer to specialist services if progress is not made in reasonable time (within 6 months of presentation). This might be a system specialty (eg, gynaecology), pain management unit or specialist urogenital pain management unit.
- Provide appropriately simplified explanations of the condition.
- Inform the patient of the resources available.

Neuropathic pain

Blair H. Smith and Mick Serpell

Keywords

- Somatosensory system.
- Anti-epileptics.

- Antidepressants.
- Leeds Assessment of Neuropathic Symptoms and Signs (LANSS).
- Allodynia.
- Hyperalgesia.
- Hyperpathia.

Objectives

- To support the diagnosis of neuropathic pain.
- To review the appropriate assessment tools that are useful in making a diagnosis.
- To facilitate an evidence-based approach to managing neuropathic pain.

Background

- The International Association for the Study of Pain defines neuropathic pain as follows:

    "… pain arising as a direct consequence of a lesion or disease affecting the somatosensory system."

- Neuropathic pain consists of a wide group of painful neurological disorders, from peripheral nerve irritation to central pain, such as that arising in stroke. There is a poor correlation between the severity of pathology and the presence of pain.

- Management of neuropathic pain remains a challenge to health care. Depression, anxiety and sleep disorders are significantly more prevalent in neuropathic pain and can cause marked suffering, disability and impaired quality of life. In primary care, it is often under-recognised and easily missed because of presentation with mixed nociceptive and idiopathic pains. The poor understanding of the complex pathogenesis of this pain by physicians often leaves patients under-treated and dissatisfied.

- All clinicians should be adequately trained to diagnose neuropathic pain in order to initiate treatment early. It is important to identify the different pain components present and treat each of them in accordance with the best available evidence.

Assessment

Pain is difficult to monitor and quantify objectively because it is a subjective phenomenon. To achieve this fully requires a combination of thorough clinical assessment and diagnostic tests.

- Focus history-taking on the characteristics of neuropathic pain (Table 3.16) and their relative contributions to the pain symptom. Importantly, symptoms should be 'neuroanatomically logical', that is their distribution should be consistent with a dermatome(s) of a diseased or damaged nerve(s) (Figure 3.5). Therefore, also clarify the presence and location of a potential cause of neuropathic pain.

- In recent years, several screening tools for distinguishing neuropathic from nociceptive pain have been validated (Table 3.16). Screening tools are not designed as diagnostic tools, but they can be useful in highlighting the need for a more detailed clinical assessment.

- The two most common tools used are the LANSS and the Douleur Neuropathique en 4 questions (DN4), which use interview questions combined with simple physical tests to achieve higher sensitivity and specificity than other screening tools that use interview-based questions only. They both have similar sensitivity and specificity, of around 85% and 90%, respectively.

Bedside examination and some important definitions

- The new criteria for stratifying neuropathic pain, as 'possible', 'probable' or 'definite', require objective evidence of either positive or negative phenomena in the somatosensory system.

- These tests are quick and easy to perform but rely on the patient's ability and willingness to co-operate.

- Include assessment of sensory, motor and autonomic phenomena in the examination in order to identify all signs of neurological dysfunction.

Modern screening tools

Questionnaires	LANNS	DN4	NPQ	Pain-DETECT	ID pain	StEP
Symptoms						
Pricking, tingling, pins and needles	x	x	x	x	x	x
Electric shocks or shooting	x	x	x	x	x	
Hot or burning	x	x	x	x	x	
Numbness		x	x	x	x	
Pain evoked by light touching	x		x	x	x	
Painful cold or freezing pain			x	x		
Clinical examination						
Brush allodynia	x	x				
Raised pin-prick threshold	x	x				x
Abnormal response to cold		x				
Hyperalgesia						x
Abnormal response to blunt pressure						x
Decreased response to vibration						x
Raised soft-touch threshold		x				
Straight-leg raising test						x

Table 3.16 Common items from several neuropathic pain screening tools – the Leeds Assessment of Neuropathic Symptoms and Signs (LANSS), Douleur Neuropathique 4 questions (DN4), the Neuropathic Pain Questionnaire (NPQ), painDETECT, ID Pain and standarized evaluation of pain (StEP). Adapted from Bennett MI *et al.* (2007) Using screening tools to identify neuropathic pain. *Pain*; **127**: 199–203. The table has been reproduced with permission of the International Association for the Study of Pain® (IASP). The table may not be reproduced for any other purpose without permission.

Dermatome chart, showing relationship between spinal nerve levels and sensory sectors in the body

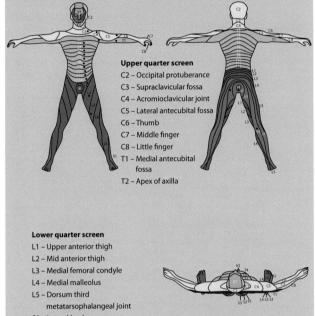

Upper quarter screen
C2 – Occipital protuberance
C3 – Supraclavicular fossa
C4 – Acromioclavicular joint
C5 – Lateral antecubital fossa
C6 – Thumb
C7 – Middle finger
C8 – Little finger
T1 – Medial antecubital fossa
T2 – Apex of axilla

Lower quarter screen
L1 – Upper anterior thigh
L2 – Mid anterior thigh
L3 – Medial femoral condyle
L4 – Medial malleolus
L5 – Dorsum third metatarsophalangeal joint
S1 – Lateral heel
S2 – Popliteal fossa
S3 – Ischial tuberosity
S5 – Perianal area

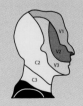

V1 – Ophthalmic division of trigeminal nerve (upper face)
V2 – Maxillary division of trigeminal nerve (mid face)
V3 – Mandibular division of trigeminal nerve (lower face)

Figure 3.5 Dermatome sectors on all diagrams are approximate because of the way sensory nerves naturally overlap of the body. Test dermatomes at dots.

- Test allodynia (pain from a non-painful stimulus) by using a light brush or piece of cotton wool over the site of pain (Figure 3.6).

- Assess hyperalgesia (an increased pain response from a mildly painful stimulus) with pin-prick testing using a 23G needle (Figure 3.6). A standardized method is needed to ensure that the same amount of pressure is applied to both the affected and the control sites.

- Also note hyperpathia (prolongation of painful sensations after the stimulus is removed) and radiation of pain.

Patient education

- Patient information is known to improve their experience and involvement with their care. It is essential for patients to be well-informed of their medical condition if they are to take an active role in its management. This is especially important for a long-term condition.

- In neuropathic pain, time spent by the doctor in discussion and explanation of symptoms and management will contribute to positive outcomes. Patient information leaflets are available from the British Pain Society, in addition to patient versions of the NICE Guidance and more recent guidance from

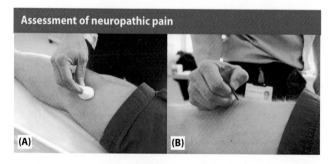

Figure 3.6 Testing for allodynia with cotton wool (A) and hyperalgesia with a blunt pin-prick (B). Taken from http/www.osceskills.com/e-learning/subjects/lower-limb-neurological-examination/.

the Scottish Intercollegiate Guideline Network. There are also websites that assist patients in working toward self-management strategies.

Drug management

NICE Clinical Guideline 173 outlines evidence-based drug management of neuropathic pain in primary care in the UK. Other countries might have similar evidence-based guidelines to support local practice but, in the absence of these, the UK NICE guidelines are accessible worldwide. For any neuropathic pain condition other than trigeminal neuralgia, first-line treatment is a choice of amitriptyline, duloxetine, gabapentin or pregabalin. If the initial treatment is ineffective or not tolerated, one of the remaining three drugs should be tried, and a further switch should be considered if the second and third drugs tried are also ineffective or not tolerated. There is no clear evidence on the benefit of combinations of these drugs. The following are suggested regimens for each drug:

- Start 10 mg of amitriptyline at night, increasing gradually to an effective dose or maximum tolerated dose (not above 75 mg). Consider alternative TCAs, such as nortriptyline. Aim for at least 25 mg of amitriptyline at night.

- Start 30 mg of duloxetine once daily, aiming to titrate to 60–120 mg/day. Consider covering the initial therapeutic period with an anti-emetic to minimize short-term side effects.

- Start 75 mg of pregabalin at night, increasing to twice daily and then gradually to an effective dose or maximum tolerated dose (no higher than 600 mg/day). Aim for at least 150 mg twice daily.

- Start 300 mg of gabapentin at night, increasing gradually, first to three times daily and then an effective dose or maximum tolerated dose (no higher than 3.6 g/day). Aim for at least 600 mg three times daily.

In the case of classical trigeminal neuralgia, carbamazepine is recommended by NICE as first-line therapy, starting at 100 mg twice daily, increasing up to 1.6 g/day if required and tolerated.

When withdrawing or switching treatment, taper down the regimen to take account of dosage and any discontinuation symptoms.

Only use tramadol if acute rescue therapy is needed and, similar to other opioids, do not use the drug for long-term treatment of neuropathic pain, unless in collaboration with a specialist. Capsaicin cream might be useful for localized neuropathic pain, particularly in people who wish to avoid, or who cannot tolerate, oral treatments.

At all stages, particularly during titration, frequent review is essential for optimal treatment. Consider early referral to a pain or neurology specialist if pain remains uncontrolled or is particularly distressing.

Side-effect management

- All systemic neuropathic analgesics can cause sedation. Other side effects, such as dizziness, dry mouth and nausea, are also common. These and rarer side effects are less likely if low doses are initiated and the dose titrated slowly upward to the maximum effective dose only if required and tolerated. Advance discussion about potential side effects is also likely to lead to greater tolerance.

- Use tramadol with caution for people on SSRI antidepressants because there is the potential for a serious serotonergic crisis.

- Combinations of antidepressants are not generally recommended. However, if a patient is already taking an SSRI or SNRI for their mood, some specialists would consider adding amitriptyline, starting at 10 mg/day but not going above 25 mg/day.

Non-drug management

- Proceed non-pharmacological approaches to treatment in parallel with drug treatment – this might include self-help, physical therapy, psychological-based therapies and multidisciplinary pain management.

- There are many studies supporting standard psychological or multidisciplinary treatment programmes in persistent pain. Only a few studies have been specifically designed for neuropathic pain. However, it would be reasonable to extrapolate the beneficial results from successful trials in generic types of persistent pain to neuropathic pain.

Management plan, including referral pathways and technological approaches

- There is a management plan for neuropathic pain recently developed for the Map of Medicine. It guides the patient's care through both primary and secondary care and is informed by the NICE guidelines. If the patient is still in pain and distress after the NICE guidance has been followed, referral to the most appropriate specialist service (pain clinic, neurology or diabetology) is recommended.

- Pain clinics offer a full multidisciplinary assessment in order to formulate the optimal management plan. They offer additional treatments for painful neuropathies, which include other more specialized drugs, injection interventions, physiotherapy, TENS and acupuncture, and training in physiotherapy and psychological self-management strategies.

- There is evidence that the use of strong opioids in post-herpetic neuralgia and some other painful neuropathies can be beneficial in relieving pain. Although NICE recommends that they only be initiated in discussion with specialists, GPs experienced in their use can be guided by the British Pain Society guidelines. In particular, it is important to screen patients for the risk of addiction and drug diversion and to agree treatment goals and monitor use.

- Drugs less widely available can be delivered by a variety of routes and might have value in treating the most resistant cases (eg, lidocaine and ketamine intravenous infusions, high-dose capsaicin skin patch [Qutenza®] and cannabinoids). Interventional pain therapies include focal diagnostic or therapeutic injections to nerves and other tissues (eg, with local anaesthetics, steroids or Botox®).

- Spinal cord stimulation is also recommended as a treatment option for adults with persistent pain of neuropathic origin in certain circumstances. Spinal drug delivery might also be appropriate for some intractable cases.

Role of the GP

- The majority of neuropathic pain can be assessed and managed within primary care.
- Be aware of the often unusual presentations and descriptions of neuropathic pain (eg, insects crawling over the skin or increased sensitivity to non-painful stimuli).
- Treat using existing pathways such as the Map of Medicine, NICE or local guidance.
- Continue to monitor drug treatment.
- Refer if diagnosis is in doubt or pain is not controlled as per pathway recommendations.
- Give the patient appropriate information on the diagnosis and self-management.

Managing co-morbidities

Amanda C de C Williams, Sarah Fox and Neil Stanley

Anxiety and depression

Supplementary videos are available in the ebook version or from the Pain Community Centre website.

Depression: Parts 1 & 2 | Sarah Fox

⊙ http://www.paincommunitycentre.org/article/depression-1-2

Time required: 60 minutes

Depression: Part 3 | Sarah Fox

⊙ http://www.paincommunitycentre.org/article/depression-3

Time required: 60 minutes

Psychosocial aspects: Depression | Owen Hughes

▶ http://www.paincommunitycentre.org/article/psychosocial-aspects-depression

Time required: 20 minutes

Keywords

- Worry.
- Loss.
- Identity.

Objectives

- Appreciate the importance of the context of pain to understand mood.
- Accept that it is normal to worry about pain until assured that it is not a serious threat.
- Recognise the importance of addressing the patient's anxieties.
- Understand the difficulties of conceptualizing depression in pain.

Background

- Acknowledging the reality of patients' pain experience is crucial.
- Most anxiety and depression in people with persistent pain is related to the pain.
- Pain is more common in depression, but pain cannot be reduced to depression.
- Depressed mood is much commoner than depression in persistent pain.

Assessment

- If the patient has pre-existing anxiety and/or depression, ask how pain affects mood and how mood affects pain.
- Anxieties are usually specific to pain and are not assessed by general anxiety questionnaires.

- Anxieties about pain usually concern the following:

  - Meaning or cause of the pain – fear of undetected disease (especially cancer in visceral pain) or of this diagnosis being withheld.

  - Inevitable worsening, with consequent loss of quality of life.

  - 'Not being able to cope' with prolonged or worse pain.

- Persistent pain causes losses of valued roles and relationships, work, leisure pursuits, satisfactions and pleasures – this is not the same as depression.

- On the PHQ-9 and other depression questionnaires, sleep disturbance, loss of pleasure in activities, low energy/activity levels, difficulty concentrating and restlessness can all be associated with pain rather than mood.

Pathway

- If depression is suspected, check for suicide risk (Table 3.17).

Diagnosis

- Diagnose depression on criteria unrelated to pain – most people with persistent pain report difficulty concentrating, loss of pleasure in activities and sleep problems, in particular.

Red flags: suicide risk
Suicidal ideation
· Ask further about plans and any attempts
· Discuss referral for psychiatric assessment
· Discuss existing possibilities for improvement in pain problem; foster hope
Suicide plans
· If involving prescribed drugs, ask about existing stocks and negotiate minimizing availability

Table 3.17

- Neither the Diagnostic and Statistical Manual (DSM; US diagnostic taxonomy) nor the International Classification of Diseases (ICD; European diagnostic taxonomy) classification is helpful in persistent pain.

Screening

- There is no adequate depression or anxiety measurement that has been developed and standardized on a population with persistent pain or chronic long-term conditions. Interpretation of existing questionnaires is therefore unreliable.

- Ask about anxieties, understanding of pain, the cause of pain (distal and proximal) and expected future. Ask about the patient's 'mental images' or 'pictures' of what is wrong or what the future holds.

- Ask about the content of mood and depressive symptoms – if sleep is disturbed, is this by pain or worry? If there is loss of pleasure in valued activities, is this because of pain or other reasons?

Management

- Management of depression includes non-pharmacological and pharmacological approaches (Table 3.18).

- Explanation of pain should include what pain is not (structural deterioration), as well as what it is (a complex mind and body system responsive to mood and activity).

- Information and patient-focussed resources, including support groups, can facilitate patients' adjustment to persistent pain.

- Treating depression is important in its own right but rarely results in significant pain relief.

- NICE Clinical Guideline 91 recommends antidepressant drugs only in patients with a history of moderate or severe depression, mild depression that complicates pain treatment or persistent subthreshold depressive symptoms.

- Addressing problems of living with pain makes it easier for the patient to manage.

- Psychological therapies are effective but only if the therapist understands pain and does not try to insist that pain is a

Good clinical practice: management of depression

- Misunderstanding a diagnosis or description can exacerbate fears: 'degenerative' (disc) to many patients means 'crumbling', causing severe disability

- Check that the patient understands the explanation and that it has not contributed to worry or hopelessness

- Reassurance that people do not 'go mad' with pain and that pain cannot be imagined into existence or abolished by willpower is valued by patients

- Consistent focus on the impact of pain on mood, sleep and day-to-day activity is important. Any treatment attempt should be discussed in terms of improvement in any or all of these, not pain relief alone

- Useful patient information, with accounts of persistent pain from patients and healthcare professionals, can be found on the HealthTalkOnline website (http://healthtalkonline.org/peoples-experiences/chronic-health-issues/chronic-pain/topics)

- Self-management information for patients who wish to work on returning toward normal activities despite pain can be found at the Pain Toolkit website (http://www.paintoolkit.org/) (p. 118)

Table 3.18

function of depression, which will distress the patient, who will usually default.

- Given the relative unlikelihood of spontaneous remission, the focus is how the patient lives a more normal life despite ongoing pain.

Treatment targets

- Improving mood.
- Improving frequency/extent of valued activities.
- Improving sleep.
- As there are no satisfactory measures of anxiety or depression in the presence of persistent pain, monitoring of progress requires either attention to ratings of specific items on questionnaires used or clinical interview.

Options

- The strongest evidence base is for cognitive-behavioural therapy, in addition to reactivation (usually by a specialist physiotherapist). Acceptance and mindfulness approaches are also effective.

- There is no evidence base at present for counselling, insight-oriented or interpersonal therapy, or general group therapy.

- Pain support groups, including expert patient programmes, can be emotionally helpful but are unlikely to help the patient to rehabilitate.

Role of the GP

- Do manage anxieties around tests and investigations, including negative results.

- Do try to provide an integrated mind and body explanation of pain.

- Do not insist that patients abandon hope of pain remitting or a miracle cure – these are not incompatible with adopting pain management methods while they wait.

- Do offer to explain the pain and associated problems to family members, who may be sceptical and unsupportive of ongoing treatment-resistant pain.

- Do address depression in the context of pain, unless it is clearly unrelated.

- If antidepressants are prescribed, clarify to the patient whether these are as analgesics or for depression (p. 89) and provide the appropriate dose.

Suicide ideation

Supplementary videos are available in the ebook version or from the Pain Community Centre website.

Suicidal ideation: Part 1 | Sarah Fox

▶ http://www.paincommunitycentre.org/article/suicidal-ideation-part-1

Time required: 30 minutes

Suicidal ideation: Part 2 | Sarah Fox

▶ http://www.paincommunitycentre.org/article/suicidal-ideation-part-2

Time required: 30 minutes

Keywords

- Suicidality.
- Passive/active suicidal ideation.
- Suicide mitigation.

Objectives

- Identify at-risk patients (awareness of specific groups).
- Assess suicidality.
- Manage suicidal ideation – suicide mitigation.

Background

- About 5000 people die from suicide each year in the UK and the WHO statistics suggest that >800,000 people die from suicide worldwide each year, which approximately corresponds to one death every 40 seconds.

- Of those who die by suicide, 25% are known to specialist mental health services – the majority of the remaining 75% will have had contact with front-line services (including primary care), a significant number within weeks of their death. NICE guidance on depression recommends that all doctors must ask patients with depression directly about suicidal ideation and intent. Studies suggest a lifetime prevalence of 30% for suicide ideation and 9.7% for suicide attempts in the general population.

- Psychotropics and pain medication are commonly used in suicide attempts by overdose (overdose accounts for 75% of attempts in patients with persistent pain).

- Male gender is associated with successful suicide, whereas female gender is associated with suicide attempts.

- Impulsivity, antisocial behaviour, domestic violence and acute family dysfunction are common risk factors (Table 3.19).

Red flags for suicide ideation and completion

Patient group	Risk
General population	3%
Major depression (in primary care, note short-duration illness carries a greater risk) NB: depression is common in persistent pain	18%
Sleep disorder	13%
Pain	Passive suicidal ideation ~20%
	Active suicidal ideation ~15%
	Current suicide plan 5%
Abdominal pain	Five-fold increase in passive suicidal ideation
	Four-fold increase in active suicidal ideation
Those of age >65 years have a higher risk for completed suicide	Also adolescents – note the influence of social media such as Youtube
Family history of suicide	First-degree relatives have greater than six-fold risk
History of suicide attempt: half of completers have attempted previously; 1 in 100 attempt survivors die by suicide within the next year	Risk 100x that of general population
Alcohol increases impulsivity and toxicity of overdose; commonly used in attempts	Suicide completers have high rates of positive blood alcohol
Substance misuse	Recreationally and/or prescribed drugs
Recently started on antidepressants	Especially SSRIs
Psychotic symptoms especially command hallucinations	Can be seen in severe depression and/or known psychotic disorder

Table 3.19 SSRI, selective serotonin reuptake inhibitor.

Assessment

The following need to be carefully explored with the patient:

* Assess the nature of suicidal thoughts, including frequency and intensity (Figure 3.7).

* Perception of the future and hopelessness.

* Planning and preparation – what is the method, how lethal? Has the patient rehearsed?

  * For patients with significant suicidal ideation, determine access to common methods of suicide, in addition to those required for the patient's specific plans, for example medicines (likely with patients who have persistent pain), firearms, vehicles or high windows/bridge/cliff/river.

  * Has the patient made any other preparations for death, for example wills, notes or given away possessions?

  * Has the patient almost acted on a plan and had to hold themselves back?

* Ability to resist acting on their thoughts of self-harm or suicide.

* Consider precipitants and exacerbating factors, in addition to factors that decrease suicidal ideation.

* Has the patient ever experienced command hallucinations?

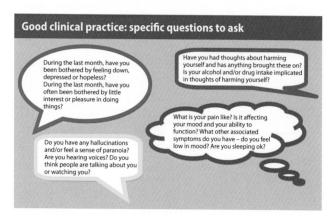

Good clinical practice: specific questions to ask

During the last month, have you been bothered by feeling down, depressed or hopeless? During the last month, have you often been bothered by little interest or pleasure in doing things?

Have you had thoughts about harming yourself and has anything brought these on? Is your alcohol and/or drug intake implicated in thoughts of harming yourself?

What is your pain like? Is it affecting your mood and your ability to function? What other associated symptoms do you have – do you feel low in mood? Are you sleeping ok?

Do you have any hallucinations and/or feel a sense of paranoia? Are you hearing voices? Do you think people are talking about you or watching you?

Figure 3.7

- Are there any mitigating factors (eg, family support)?

Examine
- Observe for signs of depression, alcohol misuse or self-harm, for example.

Test
- Assess and record capacity.
- If the patient lacks capacity:
  - Do benefits of intervention outweigh consequences of not intervening? If so, the clinician can intervene under Common Law.
- If the individual has capacity, does the person meet criteria for detention under the Mental Health Act (MHA) or local guidelines (ie, are they a danger to self and/or others)?
- MHA is uncommonly used, but about 40% of service users have avoided services for fear of being detained.

Diagnosis
- The patient admits to thoughts of self-harm – these might be passive or active, with or without intent.
- The patient admits to a plan, which might be detailed or vague.
- The patient might have rehearsed a suicide attempt.
- The patient admits to difficulty resisting ideas of self-harm.
- Evidence of self-harm.
- Evidence of a suicide attempt.

Screening
- Self-rating instruments that include one or more items on suicidal thoughts, such as the Beck Depression Inventory (BDI) and clinical face-to-face interviews have been the most widely used methods of screening:
  - Some patients feel more comfortable disclosing their suicidal thoughts using a self-rating questionnaire than discussing such information in a face-to-face interview.

- Self-rating instruments for assessing suicidal behaviours have the advantage of being standardized and are more complete and objective.

- The BDI includes a question that directly addresses suicidal ideation by instructing the patient to circle the statement that best describes the way he/she has been feeling during the past week. The response statements include the following:

  - I don't have any thoughts of killing myself.
  - I have thoughts of killing myself, but I would not carry them out.
  - I would like to kill myself.
  - I would kill myself if I had the chance.

Good clinical practice

- It might be helpful to precede initial discussions about suicidal ideation with a statement normalizing such thoughts in the setting of depression, for example*:*

  "It is common for people who are feeling sad and depressed to feel that life is not worth living or to have thoughts of ending their life. Have you had thoughts that you would … ."

- Assess and record capacity.

- NICE recommends that every person should receive a psychosocial assessment by specialist mental health professionals after an episode of self-harm.

- Overdose is a method used in 75% of attempts in patients with persistent pain. For patients at significant risk who are prescribed opiates, consider switching to skin patches that carry less risk of overdose. Prescribe limited numbers (singly or two) – this will also facilitate regular review of the patient.

- Remember that paracetamol is a commonly used drug for overdose and can be fatal in relatively small overdose.

Management

- Initial management might include triage with combined physical and mental health triage scales – urgently establish risk in a respectful way. Refer as necessary to relevant emergency or mental health teams with full information.

- Don't delay psychosocial treatment until after medical treatment.
- Avoid TCAs because of their lethal potential in the event of overdose. Safer agents include the following:
  - Fluoxetine at 20–40 mg/day.
  - Sertraline at 50–200 mg/day.
  - Venlafaxine at 75–300 mg/day.
- Elderly patients will require lower dosages.
- Patients and families should be advised that improvement might not be evident for 4–6 weeks.
- Patients might be at increased risk for suicide as their energy level improves while feelings of hopelessness and depressed mood persist. The patient should be closely followed for several weeks after the initiation of antidepressant medication.
- Because anxiety and insomnia are associated with completed suicide, these symptoms should be treated quickly, often concomitantly with antidepressant therapy.

Treatment targets

- Urgently establish physical risk and mental state in a respectful manner.
- If significant, refer to the emergency department/secondary mental health teams.
- Arrange for an appropriate chaperone if there is a risk of self-harm, especially if the patient is reluctant or distressed.
- Inform other relevant staff and organizations of the outcome of the assessment.

Options

- Risk assessment *per se* has a limited, and short-term, predictive power of a person's future risk of suicide.

- There is still 'considerable uncertainty' with regard to the most effective forms of psychosocial and physical treatments of self-harm.

- 'Cole-King Continuum' – a peer-reviewed pathway to promote 'suicide mitigation', which includes strategies such as 'risk-factor mitigation' (ie, responding to risk factors either by attempting to modify them or adding a protective factor to mitigate them).

- Applied Suicide Intervention Skills Training (ASIST) within community-based suicide prevention strategies.

Role of the GP

- Do ask about suicidal ideation – it will not increase the risk of a suicide attempt.

- Do refer to specialist services.

- Do be aware that current or recent mental health patients are more at risk (accounting for about 25% of completed suicides each year in the UK).

- Don't withdraw analgesic treatment aiming to mitigate risk, because increased pain is likely to significantly increase risk and the patient will have lost trust and might disengage, which again might increase the risk of suicidality. NICE guidelines on self-harm suggest that 43% of service users reported having avoided emergency services in the past because of previous negative experiences.

Analgesia misuse

Keywords

- Addiction.
- Dependence.
- Tolerance.

Objectives

- Awareness of types of drugs misused.
- Identify at-risk patients.

- Manage opiate misuse.
- Refer appropriately to pain and/or drug specialist services.

Background

Commonly misused analgesic or related drugs include the following:

- Opiates:

> Supplementary videos are available in the ebook version or from the Pain Community Centre website.
>
> Opiate contracts | Ian Price
>
> ⊙ http://www.paincommunitycentre.org/article/opiate-contracts
>
> Time required: 30 minutes
>
> Opiate contracts: Case studies | Ian Price
>
> ⊙ http://www.paincommunitycentre.org/article/opiate-contracts-case-studies
>
> Time required: 30 minutes

  - Particularly codeine and oxycodone.
  - Slow-release capsules might be used for injection.
  - Rarely, a fentanyl skin patch might be melted down and injected.
  - Studies report differing risks, with a spectrum ranging from <1% for short-term use in non-addicts to approximately 45% for long-term exposure in addicts.
- Benzodiazepines – might be used by pain patients to alleviate anxiety/insomnia.
- Gabapentin/pregabalin:
  - Might be used in combination recreationally (gabapentin + tramadol = 'G&T').
  - Pregabalin is increasingly used recreationally as an 'ideal psychotropic'.
  - Oral/nasal insufflation/injected.
  - Might be used to cope with opiate withdrawal.

- Ibuprofen (in combination with codeine) – available OTC.
- Ketamine:
    - 'Special K', for example.
    - Dissociative anaesthetic.
    - Hallucinogenic.
    - Might present with bladder pain.
- Cannabis.
- Some of these drugs might be used recreationally by healthy individuals.
- Polydrug use is common, as is alcohol misuse.

Assessment

- Take a full substance misuse and medication history to check for drug interactions and assist with the choice of an appropriate analgesic.
- Identify at-risk patients.
- Use the four 'C's:
    - Impaired Control over drug use.
    - Compulsive use.
    - Continued use, despite harm (Consequences).
    - Craving.

Pathway

Ask the patient about the following:

- Alcohol.
- Depression/anxiety.
- Sleep disturbance.
- Deterioration in psychosocial function (eg, work and family relationships).
- Interdose withdrawal.
- Other drug use.
- OTC medications and complementary medicine.

- Contemporaneous treatment of substance misuse (eg, methadone or Subutex®).
- Potential analgesic headaches.

Examine the patient for the following:

- Evidence of alcohol misuse.
- Pinpoint pupils, suggesting opiate use.
- Sedation/cognitive effects.
- Evidence of intravenous drug use.

Test for the following:

- Consider LFTs.
- Urine testing for drugs.

Red flags

There are several red flags for substance misuse (Table 3.20).

Diagnosis

- The patient admits to repeated use of prescription drugs outside of sanctioned medical use.
- The patient has known substance misuse problems, which might include recreational drug misuse.
- The patient's behaviour is strongly and persistently suggestive, despite previous discussion.
- The patient exhibits signs of excessive drug use.

Screening

Urine testing for opiates, for example, might be considered and/or performed by specialist services.

Good clinical practice

Documentation, including the six 'A's:

- Analgesia.
- Activity.
- Adverse effects.
- Ambiguous drug behaviours.

- Affect.
- Adequate prescription information.

Red flags: substance misuse (prescription drugs)

More predictive factors

- Multiple unsanctioned drug escalations/non-compliance; unapproved use of drug to treat other psychological symptom (eg, anxiety/insomnia)
- Persistent refusal of change in therapy, despite evidence of adverse physical or psychological effects
- Recurrent prescription 'losses', requests for early repeat prescription or problems with administration of drug (eg, a skin patch 'falling off')
- Obtaining prescription drugs from non-medical sources (eg, family or the Internet) or repeated covert acquisition from other medical sources (eg, emergency service)
- Stealing or 'borrowing' medication from other people/prescription forgery/diversion of drugs to others (giving/selling)
- Known past/continuing recreational drug use/alcohol misuse/dual diagnosis

Less predictive factors

- Occasional temporary unsanctioned dose increase (x 1–2 only), then reverts to normal prescribed dose
- Resistance to change in therapy – eg, from immediate to slow-release preparation or prescription of adjuvant medication (fear of recurrence of pain or of adverse effects)
- Reporting psychic side effects of prescribed drugs
- Drug 'hoarding', particularly during periods of reduced symptoms
- Occasional admitted acquisition of prescription drugs from other medical sources
- Requesting specific drugs, which the patient might have looked up on the Internet
- Persistent, possibly aggressive complaints about the need for higher doses to alleviate pain

Table 3.20

Management

Prescribing:

- Agree goals of treatment for persistent pain and associated symptoms (pain mitigation not eradication).

- Doses of morphine ≥120 mg/day, or equivalent, require specialist advice.

- Try to use modified-release preparations – never prescribe injections for persistent non-cancer pain.

- Evaluate requests to increase the dose carefully (consider non-pain symptoms).

- Explore inappropriate behaviour carefully and sensitively, and discuss risks of misuse of drugs, whether prescribed or recreational.

- If care is shared, be clear who is responsible for prescribing. Only one clinician should be signing repeat prescriptions. Good liaison (eg, initial telephone contact) between specialist and GP is important if opioids are prescribed for non-cancer pain generally and especially if there might be a possibility of addiction. Within a group practice, one GP should have responsibility for prescribing, with adequate arrangements for holiday cover, for example.

Treatment targets

- Separate audit criteria have been produced to support the two technology appraisals on methadone and buprenorphine (TA114) and naltrexone (TA115).

- Follow NICE guidance for the treatment of people assessed as being at risk of misusing substances. However, this is generalized guidance, unspecific to pain patients.

- Criteria 4 and 10 (CG51) relate to opportunistic brief interventions focussed on motivation offered to people with limited contact with drug services (such as those attending primary care) who have been identified as being at risk of misusing substances.

- Criterion 11 (CG51) refers to provision of information about self-help groups, which should normally be based on 12-step principles – for example, Narcotics Anonymous and Cocaine Anonymous.

- The problem with implementing these strategies in patients with persistent pain is the element of stigmatization they might feel, which is likely to be detrimental to the therapeutic relationship and might not therefore be appropriate.

Options

- There is limited published guidance for the management of patients who have persistent pain requiring opioid therapy and who are currently considered to exhibit behaviour suggestive of substance misuse or have a previous history of substance misuse.
- Tailor the therapeutic regimen to consider the risk of misuse of prescribed medication.
- This might include measures such as use of sustained-release preparations.

Role of the GP

- Do explore current and past substance use non-judgementally. If the patient refuses a transition from a short-acting to a sustained-release opioid, consider that this might not be because of addiction but psychological factors such as fear of lack of effect.
- Do consider that individual patients might respond differently to different opioids – consider appropriate treatment to alleviate associated symptoms such as depression, anxiety or insomnia.
- Do communicate with specialist services if necessary.
- Don't put patients with persistent pain in a situation whereby there is likely stigmatization. Referral to drug services for prescription drug misuse in a patient who has been prescribed these drugs to combat persistent pain might be better managed initially by pain services but, if problems persist, a further referral to specialist drug services might be considered (some specialist services run joint clinics between pain and substance misuse).

Pain and sleep (insomnia)

Keywords

- Sleep.
- Insomnia.
- Medications.

Objectives

- Appreciate the importance of sleep disturbance in the context of pain.
- Recognise the importance of addressing a patient's sleep disturbance in the successful management of pain.
- Understand the different effects that pain medications can have on sleep.

Background

- Disturbed sleep is a common co-morbidity in patients who experience either acute or persistent pain, with between 50% and 89% of patients with persistent pain demonstrating sleep disturbances.
- Many patients suffering from persistent pain experience poor sleep quality at least as significant as patients with primary insomnia.
- Difficulty sleeping ranks as one of the most reported co-morbid conditions resulting in moderate-to-severe discomfort, at nearly twice the incidence of symptoms such as depression and anxiety.
- However, although sleep disturbances might be highly prevalent in pain patients, sleep disorders in individuals with persistent pain remain under-reported, under-diagnosed and under-treated.
- Symptoms associated with sleep disturbance, such as night-time awakening and difficulty resuming sleep, result in diminished daytime functioning and ultimately emotional, physical and financial burdens.

- Sleep disturbance decreases the pain threshold and pain increases sleep disturbance, resulting in a vicious cycle, with sleep disorder and persistent pain maintaining and augmenting each other.

Assessment

Ask the patient the following initial questions:

- How do you feel during the day?
  - A sleep problem will have daytime consequences, so, if the individual feels awake and vital during the day, they might not have a problem with their sleep. If they are sleepy during the day, there is probably a problem with their sleep, so question further. NB: tiredness can be caused by many things, but sleepiness is caused by problems with sleep.
- Are you content with your sleep?
  - Answering 'no' would indicate the possibility they are suffering from insomnia – investigate further and treat, as appropriate.
- Are you excessively sleepy during the day?
  - 'Excessively sleepy' does not mean feeling sleepy at 2pm sitting in front of your computer, it means falling asleep during a conversation. Answering 'yes' would indicate the possibility of disorders such as narcolepsy, primary hypersomnia and obstructive apnoea – investigate further and refer to a sleep specialist, if appropriate.
- Does your bed-partner (or parent) complain about your sleep?
  - If answering 'yes', this indicates the possibility of suffering from a parasomnia or sleep apnoea, so investigate further and refer to a sleep specialist, if appropriate.

Diagnosis

- Because sleep disturbance is initially a subjective complaint, diagnosis must start with a careful history.
- Because there can be multiple causes of the sleep disturbance unrelated to pain, it is important that the sleep disturbance should also be assessed using criteria unrelated to pain.

- Take a sleep history (Figure 3.8) and consider asking the patient to keep a 14-day sleep diary. If this reveals a primary sleep disorder, consider referring the patient to a specialist for appropriate diagnosis and treatment.
- Although daytime sleepiness can be measured using validated questionnaires such as the Epworth Sleepiness Scale and overall sleep quality can be measured with the Pittsburgh Sleep Quality Index, no sleep questionnaire has been developed and standardized in a population with persistent pain or chronic long-term conditions.

Screening

Good clinical practice

- Assess sleep with a sleep diary and validated sleep questionnaires. Interview the bed-partner and/or caregiver about the patient's sleep.
- Review the patient's sleep hygiene and offer advice and support to improve it.
- Assess and treat patients suspected of having co-morbid sleep disturbance, for example obstructive sleep apnoea and periodic limb movements are frequent and treatable sleep disorders, and refer, as appropriate.
- Review the patient's medications and consider withdrawing medications known to disturb sleep.
- Opioids might induce or worsen sleep apnoea.
- Fully address night-time pain symptoms – use medicines with a known positive effect on sleep.
- Consider cognitive-behavioural therapy for both insomnia and pain.
- Combine non-pharmacological strategies with drug therapies, as required, for added value.
- Consider the use of hypnotics in selected patients. However, traditional hypnotic agents do not provide restorative sleep or reduce pain. Also keep in mind that benzodiazepines might worsen pain in some patients.

Sleep history

- How often do you have trouble sleeping and how long have you had the problem?
- When do you go to bed and get up on workdays and days off?
- How long does it take you to fall asleep, how often and why do you wake up at night, and how long does it take to fall back asleep?
- Do you snore loudly and often or wake up gasping or feeling out of breath?
- How refreshed do you feel when you wake up, and how tired do you feel during the day?
- How often do you doze off or have trouble staying awake during routine tasks, especially driving?
- Do you worry about falling asleep, staying asleep or getting enough sleep?
- What do you eat or drink, and do you take medicines before going to bed?
- What routine do you follow before going to bed?
- What are the noise level, lighting and temperature like where you sleep?
- What distractions, such as a television or computer, are in your bedroom?

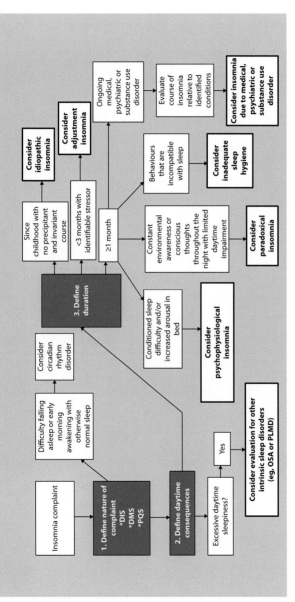

Figure 3.8 DIS, difficulty initiating sleeping; DMS, difficulty maintaining sleeping; OSA, obstructive sleep apnoea; PLMD, periodic limb movement disorder; PQS, poor quality sleep. Algorithm for evaluating insomnia according to the International Classification of Sleep Disorders, second edition. Adapted from Tripathi M and Vibha D (2011) Approach to a patient with insomnia. *Indian J Sleep Med* **6:**1-6.

Management

Concurrent management of disturbed sleep and pain in patients with persistent pain is advisable, and neuropathic pain guidelines specifically recommend the assessment of sleep in the management of pain patients.

Treatment targets

- Improve the quality of sleep.
- Treat other co-morbid sleep problems, which might disturb sleep – for example, obstructive sleep apnoea and periodic limb movement disorder.
- Reduction of anxiety/depression.
- Improve patients' functionality and quality of life.
- Assessment of medications and their effects on sleep (Table 3.21).

Role of the GP

- Do take a complaint of poor sleep seriously – it requires more than a prescription of amitriptyline (which is a sedative and does not necessarily improve sleep quality).
- Do ask your patients about their sleep and how it affects them.
- Do treat any sleep problems appropriately, according to the evidence base, whether they are related to pain or not.

Effects of various medications used in the treatment of pain on sleep

Drug/drug class	Effects on sleep	Overall effect on sleep
NSAIDs (aspirin and ibuprofen)	Increase SOL and awakenings Decrease SWS	–
Opioids	Decrease SWS and REM sleep Increase nocturnal wake time (prolonged sleep latency and increased awakenings) Might induce or worsen sleep apnoeas	–
Tramadol	Increases stage 2 sleep Decreases SWS and REM	–
TCAs	Decrease REM sleep and nocturnal awakenings Possibly increase SWS	–/+
SSRIs	Increase SOL and stages 1 and 2 sleep Reduces REM sleep and SWS	–
SNRIs	Increase stages 1 and 2 sleep and SOL Reduces REM sleep and SWS	–
Carbamazepine	Increases stages 1 and 2 NREM sleep and depresses REM sleep Reduces SOL	–/+
Gabapentin	Increases SWS	+
Pregabalin	Increases SWS Reduces arousals/awakenings Decreases SOL	+
Cognitive-behavioural therapy (insomnia)	Reduces SOL Increases sleep duration	+

Table 3.21 NREM, non-rapid eye movement; NSAID, non-steroidal anti-inflammatory drugs; REM, rapid eye movement; SOL, sleep-onset latency; SNRI serotonin–norepinephrine reuptake inhibitor; SSRI, selective serotonin reuptake inhibitor; SWS, slow-wave sleep; TCA, tricyclic antidepressant.

Self-management

Frances Cole

Keywords

- Person-centred assessment.
- Self-efficacy.
- Collaboration.
- Enabling.
- Core skill development.

Objectives

- To examine the multidimensional impact of persistent pain and why self-management is vitally important.
- To describe the principles of self-management.
- To discuss the main barriers to effective self-management.
- To consider the role of acceptance.

Background

- The individual with long-term pain requires robust self-management knowledge, skills and resources to sustain confidence in coping with its challenging, detrimental cognitive, emotional, behavioural, physical and life consequences.
- The average annual consultation time individuals with pain conditions receive from healthcare professionals is 3 h, so it is crucial that individuals cope effectively with pain in their everyday life.

- Pain has a multidimensional impact on an individual's health function, with many changeable aspects through self-management, the commonest benefits being the following:

  - Improvement of physical fitness.

  - Improvement of pain relief.

  - Addressing sleep disturbance.

  - Improvement of mood changes, including depression, anxiety, pain-related stress and anger.

Principles of self-management
Frances Cole

> "Self-care or self-management refers to activities individuals, families and communities undertake with the intention of enhancing health, preventing, disease, limiting illness and restoring health. These activities are derived from knowledge and skills from the pool of both professionals' and patients' experiences. They are undertaken by individuals on their own behalf, either separately or in participative collaboration with professionals."
>
> *WHO, 1983*

Key steps for patients with or without clinician or non-clinician support (ie, by themselves):

- Identifying the impact of pain using a person-centred assessment, with a tool like the Health Needs Assessment or vicious circle of pain (Figures 4.1 and 4.2).

- Identifying the patient's current priorities for change in self-management and clinical management approaches.

- Understanding crucial knowledge, learning and using key skills, and patients reviewing progress themselves using self-confidence to cope with pain, health function or wellbeing measures.

- Knowing how to access further information, resources and support over time.

Health Needs Assessment (HNA) for persistent pain

Changing how the pain affects your life

Pain can affect peoples' lives in many ways. This questionnaire lists some of the problems and difficulties due to longstanding pain.

Please help us understand the main problems **at present** that you feel are important to improve your quality of the life and self manage with more confidence.

Step 1: Please tick ✓ the boxes below related to your needs now, and then complete **Step 2.**

Name: **Date of birth:**

Do you have any problems or difficulties with:

1. ☐ Walking or moving about
2. ☐ Lack of fitness and energy
3. ☐ Balance or recurrent falls
4. ☐ Side effects or other problems with current pain medication (eg, tablets, etc)
5. ☐ Pain relief
6. ☐ Understanding why longstanding pain occurs
7. ☐ An unhelpful pattern of activity of doing too much, getting more pain, then doing too little
8. ☐ Eating the right sort of foods
9. ☐ Disturbed sleep
10. ☐ Managing mood changes of depression, anger, anxiety or worry
11. ☐ Tiredness or lack of energy
12. ☐ Relationship difficulties, with partner, family, work, etc
13. ☐ Sex life
14. ☐ Remaining in work or returning to work and/or training
15. ☐ Financial or money difficulties
16. ☐ Current legal claim linked with the pain problem
17. ☐ Concerns about your carer/partner, their health or other problems
18. ☐ Other difficulties that you feel are important to change, for example, concerns about housing, hobbies, leisure or social events with friends or visiting the church of mosque. Please describe here

----

Step 2: If you ticked more than **three areas of your life**, please circle the **three** most important to change at present.

Thank you for helping us to understand your main needs due to pain.

Figure 4.1

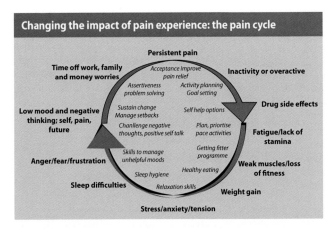

Figure 4.2 Reproduced with permission from http://www.paintoolkit.org/.

Self-management knowledge and skills address three aspects:

- Enabling the individual to comprehensively understand their condition(s), the ways it affects the body and mind, and its prognosis.

- Patients' collaboration with clinicians and non-clinicians enables them to explore how they can positively help themselves reduce the impact of pain – for example, through better knowledge of their condition(s) so they can accurately interpret body symptoms rather than take a catastrophic view.

- Patients becoming skilled in managing daily activities, thus keeping in balance the pain experienced, fatigue, mood changes and other symptoms, and so lessening the impact of pain.

The general principles of self-management are as follows:

- Core skills are most valued (Figure 4.2, italicized font). The application of these skills in everyday life leads to increased self-confidence to cope and function well, despite the pain (self-efficacy). These coping strategies or skills can deal more specifically with pain symptoms and minimize pain-related distress and disability. Also, these strategies enable the individual to move to a state of mind in which they are aware of the pain, become more accepting of the pain and not to try to avoid or actively change it.

- Self-management on the basis of cognitive-behavioural principles has an evidence base indicating beneficial changes in pain experienced, cognitive coping in positive ways and reduction in behavioural expressions of pain.

- Recent work with those engaging in self-management through pain management groups found four key aspects effect benefits:

  - Peer support reduces isolation.

  - Communication self-advocacy and with healthcare professionals, "You should not be feeling like this", vs the empathetic environment of the pain management programme, "You understand and see my distress".

  - Knowledge – information on tools, pain physiology and why pain persists.

  - Past and present self-identity – that is, the dichotomy between past and present selves; increased confidence, self-management tools and facilitated recovery of past and preferred self concepts.

- Types of self-management are varied, including information leaflets, websites, peer-support groups, email discussion and formal pain management programmes, with and without psychological interventions, either on an individual basis, on a group basis or computer-based. The type of self-management approach depends on the individual, their preferred method of learning, their preference to participate in group programmes and whether they have sensory or other disabilities or literacy issues.

- Timing of self-management approaches should be much earlier than is currently happening in routine clinical practice, in which it is usually years rather than months from the onset of pain. Feedback from patients shows it is needed within weeks of the onset of pain to facilitate positive coping strategies and attitudes to maintain health function and reduce disability and distress. It is crucial to enable patient access to self-management skills and resources much earlier because it is more beneficial to health.

Common barriers to engagement in self-management are as follows:

- Patient barriers:
  - Lack of acceptance of the long-term nature of the pain condition.
  - Fear of pain-related movement (kiniesophobia).
  - Mood change linked specifically to pain (depression, anxiety and anger).
  - Life events (change or loss of work or status, financial or housing difficulties, relationship breakdown, family illness or bereavements).
  - Language, cultural, literacy or dyslexia difficulties.
  - Adopting a 'sick role'.
  - Drug or alcohol problems.
  - Mental health problems (bipolar disorder, psychosis or dementia).
  - Loss and lack of adjustment.
  - Other co-morbidities (obesity, diabetes or heart disease).
- Clinician barriers:
  - Persistent focus on a biomedical approach to pain rather than a biopsychosocial model.
  - Concentration on a cure for pain rather than management.
  - Inadequate consultation skills to motivate and collaborate with the patient and their person-centred agenda.
  - Failure to identify depression, anxiety or anger mood changes.
  - Inadequate education on the true nature of persistent pain.
  - Lack of skills and tools to engage patients in self-management choices and decisions, to enable them adjust to the impact of their condition.
  - Insufficient consultation time.
  - Lack of clarity about changing roles and partnership between clinicians and patients.

Acceptance and letting go of the futile search for a cure or total pain relief is a major obstacle to enabling self-management and lessening pain-related distress. Consistent messages are required from clinicians that pain is a long-term condition, with a shift from biomedical to person-centred approaches and linking self-management resources, thus contributing to the process of acceptance.

Shared decision-making is a crucial part of self-management and requires patients to be willing to engage actively. Clinicians should understand their patients' values and preferences and be skilled in risk communication and the use of aids to facilitate patient communication and questions.

What is a pain self-management programme? A simple guide for GPs and patients from a patient's perspective

Peter Moore

- With ever-increasing numbers of patients living with pain and long-term health conditions, self-management is becoming even more important.

- Learning to self-manage is like learning any other skill. For example, learning to drive a car can take time, practise and encouragement, and learning to self-manage pain and a health condition is similar.

- 'Self-management' must not be confused with 'self-care':
  - Self-care is carrying out everyday care, washing and brushing teeth, for example.
  - Self-management is taking action and patients working in partnership with their healthcare teams (supported self-management). It also promotes 'self-efficacy'.

- Patients will also need a selection of tools (skills) to self-manage their pain and long-term health condition and *The Pain Toolkit* could be useful to support them to do this.

- *The Pain Toolkit* is a simple information booklet that can provide patients with handy tips and skills to support them along the way to manage their pain. It is not meant to be the last word in pain self-management but rather a handy guide to help them get started.

- Many healthcare professionals now use *The Pain Toolkit* to support their patients to start the process to pain self-management (p. 127).

- Patients who are good pain self-managers have the following qualities:

  - Good listeners.
  - Clear communicators.
  - Work in partnership with others – teamwork.
  - Resource finders.
  - Monitor their condition and report back to their healthcare team.
  - Outward-focussed.
  - Problem-solvers.
  - Maintain physical and emotional wellbeing.
  - Partners in care.
  - Confident.

Role of the GP

- Be aware that persistent pain is a long-term condition.
- Provide patients with consistent messages about their pain.
- Be confident in providing patients with persistent pain self-management skills at an early stage after diagnosis and support them through their journey.
- Sign-post patients to other agencies and information sources.

Further reading

American Academy of Sleep Medicine (2005) *The International Classification of Sleep Disorders*, 2nd edition. Rochester: American Sleep Disorders Association.

Argoff CE (2007) The Coexistence of Neuropathic Pain, Sleep, and Psychiatric Disorders: A Novel Treatment Approach. *Clin J Pain* **23:**15–22.

Arnold LM *et al.* (2007) Gabapentin in the treatment of fibromyalgia: a randomized, double-blind, placebo-controlled, multicenter trial. *Arthritis Rheum* **56:**1336–44.

Arnold LM *et al.* (2012) FibroCollaborative. A framework for fibromyalgia management for primary care providers. *Mayo Clin Proc* **87:**488–96.

Arthritis Care. http://www.arthritiscare.org.uk (accessed 7th March 2014).

Arthritis Research Campaign. http://www.arc.org.uk (accessed 7th March 2014).

Atherton K *et al.* (2009) Vitamin D and chronic widespread pain in a white middle-aged British population: evidence from a cross-sectional population survey. *Ann Rheum Dis* **68:**817–22.

Audit criteria for methadone (TA114) and naltrexone (TA115). http://www.nice.org.uk/nicemedia/live/11812/38215/38215.doc (accessed 9th May 2012).

BackCare. http://www.backcare.org.uk (accessed 7th March 2014).

Baranidharan G *et al.* (2012) Lumbar spine interventions. In: *Spinal interventions in pain management: Oxford specialists handbook in pain medicine.* (Eds: K Simpson *et al.*) Oxford: Oxford University Press; pp 37–70.

Battersby M *et al.* (2010) Twelve evidence-based principles for implementing self-management support in primary care. *Jt Comm J Qual Patient Saf* **36:**561–70.

Beck AT *et al.* (1996) BDI-II. http://www.tandfonline.com/doi/abs/10.1207/s15327752jpa6703_13#.U6Gn0yjTzcg (accessed 3rd July 2014).

Bennett M (2001) The LANSS pain scale: the Leeds Assessment of Neuropathic Symptoms and Signs. *Pain* **92:**147–57.

Bennett MI *et al.* (2006) Can pain can be more or less neuropathic? Comparison of symptom assessment tools with ratings of certainty by clinicians. *Pain* **122:**289–94.

Bennett MI *et al.* (2007) Using screening tools to identify neuropathic pain. *Pain* **127:**199–203.

Bogduk N and Merskey H (1994) *Classification of chronic pain: descriptions of chronic pain syndromes and definitions of pain terms*, 2nd edition. Seattle: IASP Press.

Bogduk N *et al.* (2009) A narrative review of lumbar medial branch neurotomy for the treatment of back pain. *Pain Med* **10:**1035–45.

Breathworks mindfulness-based pain management. http://www.breathworks-mindfulness.co.uk (accessed 7th March 2014).

Breivik H *et al.* (2006) Survey of chronic pain in Europe: prevalence, impact on daily life, and treatment. *Eur J Pain* **10:**287–333.

Bridges stroke self-management. http://www.bridges-stroke.org.uk/self_management.php (accessed 7th March 2014).

Bridges S (2011) Chapter 9: Chronic Pain. In: *Health Survey England*, Volume 1. https://catalogue.ic.nhs.uk/publications/public-health/surveys/heal-surv-eng-2011/HSE2011-Ch9-Chronic-Pain.pdf (accessed 7th March 2014).

Brief Pain Inventory. http://www.mdanderson.org/education-and-research/departments-programs-and-labs/departments-and-divisions/symptom-research/symptom-assessment-tools/bpisf.pdf (accessed 7th March 2014).

British National Formulary. http://www.bnf.org (accessed 7th March 2014).

British Pain Society: A professional alliance of those involved in pain and its management. http://www.britishpainsociety.org.uk (accessed 27th September 2012).

British Pain Society (2005) The use of drugs beyond licence in palliative care and pain management. http://www.britishpainsociety.org/book_usingdrugs_main.pdf (accessed 22 January 2014).

British Pain Society (2007) Pain and substance misuse: improving the patient experience. http://www.britishpainsociety.org/book_drug_misuse_main.pdf (accessed 7th March 2014).

British Pain Society (2007) Recommended guidelines for pain management programmes for adults. http://www.britishpainsociety.org/book_pmp_main.pdf (accessed 3rd July 2014).

British Pain Society (2010) Opioids for persistent pain: a summary of guidance on good practice from the British Pain Society. http://www.britishpainsociety.org/book_opioid_main.pdf (accessed 3rd July 2014).

British Pain Society (2010) Opioids for persistent pain: information for patients. http://www.britishpainsociety.org/book_opioid_patient.pdf (accessed 22 January 2014).

British Pain Society (2010) *Understanding and Managing Pain*. London: BPS.

British Pain Society's Map of Medicine Pathways. http://bps.mapofmedicine.com/evidence/bps/index.html (accessed 11 March 2014).

BUPA for specific pelvic pain information. http://www.bupa.co.uk/individuals/health-information (accessed 7th March 2014).

Burckhardt C *et al.* (2005) *Guideline for the Management of Fibromyalgia Syndrome Pain in Adults and Children*. Chicago: American Pain Society.

Burton AK *et al.* (1999) Information and Advice to Patients With Back Pain Can Have a Positive Effect: A Randomized Controlled Trial of a Novel Educational Booklet in Primary Care. *Spine* **24:**2484–91.

Busch A *et al.* Exercise for treating fibromyalgia syndrome. Cochrane Database Syst Rev. 2003;3:CD003786.

Buysse DJ *et al.* (1989). The Pittsburgh Sleep Quality Index (PSQI): A new instrument for psychiatric research and practice. *Psychiatr Res* **28:**193–213.

Canadian Guideline for Safe and Effective use of Opioids for chronic non-cancer pain (2010). http://nationalpaincentre.mcmaster.ca/documents/opioid_guideline_part_a_v4_5.pdf (accessed 7th March 2014).

Carville SF *et al.* (2008) EULAR evidence-based recommendations for the management of fibromyalgia syndrome. *Ann Rheum Dis* **67:**536–41.

Chaparro LE *et al.* (2013) Opioids compared to placebo or other treatments for chronic low-back pain. Cochrane library.

Chronic Pain Scotland: Living well with chronic pain. http://chronicpainscotland.org/patients-area/living-well-with-chronic-pain/ (accessed 19 December 2013).

Cole F *et al.* (2005) *Overcoming Chronic Pain*. London: Constable Robinson.

Cole-King A and Lepping P (2010) Suicide mitigation: time for a more realistic approach. *Br J Gen Pract* **60:**e1–e3.

Cole-King Suicide Mitigation. http://www.connectingwithpeople.org/sites/default/files/SuicideMitigationInPrimaryCareFactsheet_0612.pdf (accessed 2nd April 2014).

Connecting with People: Training for Primary Care Teams in Suicide and Self Harm Awareness and Suicide Risk Response. http://www.wales.nhs.uk/sites3/Documents/749/Connecting%20with%20People%20Positive%20Choices%20Primary%20Care%20Overview%20-%20Feb%202010.pdf (accessed 7th March 2014).

Controlled Drugs in Primary Care, 2nd edition (2005). http://www.controlleddrugs.org (accessed 7th March 2014).

Conversion tables (Wales, UK). http://www.wales.nhs.uk/sites3/Documents/814/OpiateConversionDoses%5BFinal%5DNov2010.pdf (accessed 7th March 2014).

Coulter A and Ellins J (2006) Patient-focused interventions: A review of the evidence (QQUIP). http://www.health.org.uk/ (accessed 24th September 2014).

Crews KR *et al.* (2014) Clinical Pharmacogenetics Implementation Consortium Guidelines for Cytochrome P450 2D6 Genotype and Codeine Therapy: 2014 Update. *Clin Pharmacol Ther* **95:**376–82.

Crofford LJ *et al.* (2008) Fibromyalgia relapse evaluation and efficacy for durability of meaningful relief (FREEDOM): a 6-month, double-blind, placebo-controlled trial with pregabalin. *Pain* **136:**419–31.

Croft P (2010) Aches and pains in primary care: stay positive but critical. *Br J Gen Pract* **60:**79–80.

Daniel HC *et al.* (2008) Comparison of psychological and physical function in neuropathic pain and nociceptive pain: Implications for cognitive behavioral pain management programs. *Eur J Pain* **12:**731–41.

Dansie EJ and Turk DC (2013) Assessment of patients with chronic pain. *Br J Anaesthesiol* **111:**19–25.

Davies KA *et al.* (2008) Restorative sleep predicts the resolution of chronic widespread pain: results from the EPIFUND study. *Rheumatology (Oxford)* **47:**1809–13.

Davis L *et al.* (2007) Modern combined oral contraceptives for pain associated with endometriosis. Cochrane Database Syst Rev; CD001019.

De C Williams AC and Johnson M (2011) Pain not a 'medically unexplained symptom'. *Br J Gen Prac* **61:**638–9.

Denk F *et al.* (2014) Pain vulnerability: a neurobiological perspective. *Nat Neurosci* **17**:192–200.

Department of Health (2005) *Self Care—a real choice: self care support a practical option.* London: DOH.

Department of Health Musculoskeletal Framework (2006). http://webarchive.national-alarchives.gov.uk/20130107105354/http://www.dh.gov.uk/prod_consum_dh/groups/dh_digitalassets/@dh/@en/documents/digitalasset/dh_4138412.pdf (accessed 22 January 2014).

Depression Alliance. http://www.depressionalliance.org (accessed 7th March 2014).

Dickman A and Simpson K (2008) *Chronic Pain.* Oxford: Oxford University Press.

Dimsdale JE *et al.* (2007) The effect of opioids on sleep architecture. *J Clin Sleep Med* **3**:33–6.

D'Mello R and Dickenson AH (2008) Spinal cord mechanisms of pain. *Br J Anaesth* **101**:8–16.

DoloTest. http://www.dolotest.com (accessed 7th March 2014).

Donaldson L (2009) 150 years of the Annual Report of the Chief Medical Officer: On the state of public health 2008. London: Department of Health. http://webarchive.national-archives.gov.uk/20130107105354/http://www.dh.gov.uk/en/Publicationsandstatistics/Publications/AnnualReports/DH_096206 (accessed 25th March 2014).

Drewes AM and Arendt-Nielsen L (2001) Pain and sleep in medical diseases: interactions and treatment possibilities (A review). *Sleep Research Online* **4**:67–76.

Dworkin RH *et al.* (2007) Pharmacologic management of neuropathic pain: evidence-based recommendations. *Pain* **132**:237–51.

Eccleston C *et al.* (2009) Psychological therapies for the management of chronic pain (excluding headache) in adults. Cochrane Library, Issue 2.

Engel GL (1977) The need for a new medical model: a challenge for biomedicine. *Science* **196**:129–36.

Engel GL (1980) The clinical application of the biopsychosocial model. *Am J Psychiatry* **137**:535–44.

Engeler D *et al.* (2012) EAU guidelines on chronic pelvic pain. http://www.uroweb.org/guidelines/online-guidelines/ (accessed 7th March 2014).

Erowid (drug experiences). https://www.erowid.org/experiences/exp_front.shtml (accessed 7th March 2014).

Expert patients programme. http://www.expertpatients.co.uk (accessed 7th March 2014).

Fibromyalgia Association UK. http://www.fibromyalgia-associationuk.org (accessed 7th March 2014).

Fibromyalgia syndrome: management in primary care; Arthritis Research UK. http://www.arthritisresearchuk.org/~/media/Files/Education/Hands-On/HO07-Autumn-2010.ashx (accessed 7th March 2014).

Finnerup N *et al.* (2005) Algorithm for neuropathic pain treatment: an evidence based proposal. *Pain* **118**:289–305.

Flockhart DA (2007) Drug Interactions: Cytochrome P450 Drug Interaction Table. Indiana University School of Medicine. http://medicine.iupui.edu/clinpharm/ddis/clinical-table/ (accessed 7th March 2014).

Freynhagen R *et al.* (2006) PainDETECT: a new screening questionnaire to identify neuropathic components in patients with back pain. *Curr Med Res Opin* **22:**1911–20.

Gatchel RJ *et al.* (2007) The biopsychosocial approach to chronic pain: Scientific advances and future directions. *Psychol Bull* **133:**581–624.

Ghahreman A *et al.* (2010) The efficacy of transforaminal injection of steroids for the treatment of lumbar radicular pain. *Pain Med* **11:**1149–68.

Goldenberg D *et al.* (1996) Randomized, double-blind crossover trial of fluoxetine and amitriptyline in the treatment of fibromyalgia. *Arthritis Rheum* **39:**1852–9.

Goldenberg DL *et al.* (2004) Management of fibromyalgia syndrome. *JAMA* **292:**2388–95.

Goodfellow C *et al.* (2013) "We know it works but why" a qualitative study of participants after pain management programme. LH.CALM@nhs.net

Gray P (2008) Acute neuropathic pain: diagnosis and treatment. *Curr Opin Anaesthesiol* **21:**590–5.

Gupta A *et al.* (2007) The role of psychosocial factors in predicting the onset of chronic widespread pain: results from a prospective population based study. *Rheumatology (Oxford)* **46:**666–71.

Gupta S and Haider S (2012) Focal Back Pain and its Management. In: *Symptom oriented pain management*. (Eds: Baheti DK *et al.*) New Dehli: Jaypee Brothers Medical Publishers; pp 98–109.

Haanpaa ML *et al.* (2009) Assessment of neuropathic pain in primary care. *Am J Med* **122(10 Suppl):**S13–21.

Harden H and Cohen M (2003) Unmet needs in the management of neuropathic pain. *J Pain Symptom Manage* **25(Suppl 5):**S12–7.

Häuser W *et al.* (2009) Treatment of fibromyalgia syndrome with gabapentin and pregabalin--a meta-analysis of randomized controlled trials. *Pain* **145:**69–81.

Häuser W *et al.* (2012) The role of antidepressants in the management of fibromyalgia syndrome: a systematic review and meta-analysis. *CNS Drugs* **26:**297–307.

Hawton KKE *et al.* (1999) Psychosocial and pharmacological treatments for deliberate self harm. Cochrane Database of Systematic Reviews, Issue 3. Art. No.: CD001764. DOI: 10.1002/14651858.CD001764

Health Survey England (2011). http://www.natcen.ac.uk/series/health-survey-for-england (accessed 7th March 2014).

Health Talk Online. http://www.healthtalkonline.org (accessed 7th March 2014).

Hicks JK *et al.* (2013) Clinical Pharmacogenetics Implementation Consortium Guideline for CYP2D6 and CYP2C19 Genotypes and Dosing of Tricyclic Antidepressants. *Clin Pharmacol Ther* **93:**402–8.

Holden AV *et al.* (1984) *The Neurobiology of pain*. Manchester: Manchester University Press.

Hughes G *et al*. (2006) The impact of a diagnosis of fibromyalgia on health care re-source use by primary care patients in the UK: an observational study based on clinical practice. *Arthritis Rheum* **54:**177–83.

International Pain Summit Of The International Association For The Study Of Pain (2011) Declaration of Montréal: declaration that access to pain management is a fundamental human right. *J Pain Palliat Care Pharmacother* **25:**29–31.

Jensen TS *et al*. (2011) A new definition of neuropathic pain. *Pain* **152:**2204–5.

Johns MW (1991) A new method for measuring daytime sleepiness: The Epworth Sleepiness Scale. *Sleep* **14:**540–5.

Kaplan KH *et al*. (1993) The impact of a meditation-based stress reduction program on fibromyalgia. *Gen Hosp Psychiatry* **15:**284–9.

Keele STarT Back Tool for back pain. http://www.keele.ac.uk/sbst (accessed 7th March 2014).

Kirklees Persistent Pain. http://www.kirkleespersistentpain.com/ (accessed 7th March 2014).

Kroenke K *et al*. (2001) A brief measure for assessing generalised anxiety disorder: the GAD-7. *Arch Intern Med* **16:**606–13.

Kroenke K *et al*. (2001) The PHQ-9: validity of a brief depression severity measure. *J Gen Intern Med* **16:**606–13.

Kung S *et al*. (2013) Comparing the Beck Depression Inventory-II (BDI-II) and Patient Health Questionnaire (PHQ-9) depression measures in an integrated mood disorders practice. *J Affective Disorders* **145:**341–3.

Langley P *et al*. (2010) The impact of pain on labor force participation, absenteeism and presenteeism in the European Union. *J Med Econ* **13:**662–72.

Langley P *et al*. (2010) The societal impact of pain in the European Union: health-related quality of life and healthcare resource utilization. *J Med Econ* **13:**571–81.

Living with chronic pain DVD / CD by Neil Berry. http://www.paincd.org.uk/ (accessed 7th March 2014).

Main CJ and George SZ (2011) Psychologically informed practice for management of low back pain: future directions in practice and research. *Phys Ther* 91:820–4.

Management of patients with physical and psychological problems in primary care (2009). http://www.rcgp.org.uk/pdf/corp_management_of_patients_with_physical_and_psychological_problems_in_primary_care.pdf (accessed 7th March 2014).

Manchikanti L *et al*. (2013) An update of comprehensive evidence-based guidelines for interventional techniques in chronic spinal pain. Part II: Guidance and recommendations. *Pain Physician* **16:**S49–S283.

Marjoribanks J *et al*. (2010) Nonsteroidal anti-inflammatory drugs for dysmenorrhoea, Cochrane Database of Systematic Reviews. Chichester: John Wiley & Sons.

Mark A *et al*. (2008) Pain and suicidal thoughts, plans and attempts in the United States. *Gen Hosp Psychiatry* **30:**521–7.

McCaffery M and Beebe A (1989) *Pain: clinical manual for nursing practice*. St Louis: C.V. Mosby.

McIntosh G and Hall H (2008) Low back pain (acute). *Clin Evid* **10:**1102–32.

McNicol ED *et al.* (2013) Opioids for neuropathic pain. Cochrane library.

ME Association. http://www.meassociation.org.uk (accessed 7th March 2014).

Medial branch block injections and radiofrequency denervation for low back pain of lumbar facet origin. Prepared by the British Pain Society and Faculty of Pain Medicine of the Royal College of Anaesthetists (In Press).

Menefee LA *et al.* (2000) Sleep disturbance and nonmalignant chronic pain: a comprehensive review of the literature. *Pain Med* **1:**156–72.

Mental Health Act (2005). http://www.legislation.gov.uk/ukpga/2007/12/contents (accessed 2nd May 2012).

Mental Health Act Scotland (2003). http://www.scotland.gov.uk/Resource/Doc/55971/0015983.pdf (accessed 8th February 2012).

Migraine Trust. http://www.migrainetrust.org (accessed 7th March 2014).

MIND confidential help and advice. http://www.mind.org.uk (accessed 7th March 2014).

Moore RA *et al.* (2009) Pregabalin for acute and chronic pain in adults, Cochrane Database of Systematic Reviews. Chichester: John Wiley & Sons.

Moore RA *et al.* (2011) Gabapentin for chronic neuropathic pain and fibromyalgia in adults, Cochrane Database of Systematic Reviews. Chichester: John Wiley & Sons.

Moore RA *et al.* (2014) The costs and consequences of adequately managed chronic non-cancer pain and chronic neuropathic pain. *Pain Pract* **14:**79–94.

Morley S *et al.* (1999) Systematic review and meta-analysis of randomised controlled trails of cognitive behaviour therapy and behaviour therapy for chronic pain in adults excluding headache. *Pain* **80:**1–13.

Mourao AF *et al.* (2010) Generalised musculoskeletal pain syndromes. *Best Practice & Research Clinical Rheumatology* **24:**829–40.

Moodjuice: a site designed to help individuals think about emotional problems and work towards solving them. http://www.moodjuice.scot.nhs.uk/mildmoderate/ChronicPain.asp (accessed 19 December 2013).

Multiple Sclerosis Society. http://www.mssociety.org.uk (accessed 7th March 2014).

National Institute for Health and Clinical Excellence (2004) CG16 - Self-harm: the short-term physical and psychological management and secondary prevention of self-harm in primary and secondary care. London: NICE. http://www.nice.org.uk/CG016 (accessed 7th March 2014).

National Institute for Health and Clinical Excellence (2007) CG51 - Drug misuse: Psychosocial interventions. London: NICE. http://www.nice.org.uk/guidance/cg51/resources/cg51-drug-misuse-psychosocial-interventions-full-guideline2 (accessed 20th August 2014).

National Institute for Health and Clinical Excellence (2008) TA159: Spinal Cord Stimulation for Chronic Pain of Neuropathic or Ischaemic Origin. London: NICE.

National Institute for Health and Clinical Excellence (2009) Management of long-term sickness and incapacity for work. Public Health Guidance 19. London: NICE. http://www.nice.org.uk/nicemedia/live/11779/43545/43545.pdf (accessed 22 January 2014).

National Institute for Health and Clinical Excellence (2009) CG90 - Depression in adults: The treatment and management of depression in adults. London: NICE. http://www.nice.org.uk/CG90 (accessed 7th March 2014).

National Institute for Health and Clinical Excellence (2009) CG91 - Depression in adults with a chronic physical health problem. London: NICE. http://guidance.nice.org.uk/CG91/NICEGuidance/pdf/English (accessed 25th March 2014).

National Institute for Health and Clinical Excellence (2013) CG173 - Neuropathic Pain—Pharmacological Management: The pharmacological management of neuropathic pain in adults in non-specialist settings. London: NICE. http://guidance.nice.org.uk/CG173 (accessed 19 December 2013).

National Institute for Health and Clinical Excellence (2014) CG177 - Osteoathritis: care and management in adults. London: NICE.

'Neuropathic pain' (PDF) from Patient UK. http://www.patient.co.uk (accessed 7th March 2014).

'Neuropathic pain' (PDF) from the Brain and Spine Foundation. http://www.brainandspine.org.uk (accessed 7th March 2014).

NHS Choices. http://www.nhs.uk (accessed 7th March 2014).

Noble M *et al.* (2010) Long-term opioid management for chronic noncancer pain, Cochrane Database of Systematic Reviews. Chichester: John Wiley & Sons.

Nüesch E *et al.* (2009) Oral or transdermal opioids for osteoarthritis of the knee or hip. Cochrane library.

Onen SH *et al.* (2005) How pain and analgesics disturb sleep. *Clin J Pain* **21:**422–31.

Opioid-equivalent tables. http://endoflife.stanford.edu/M11_pain_control/equivalency_table.html (accessed 7th March 2014).

Opioids for Persistent Pain; Good Practice. The British Pain Society, the Faculty of Pain Medicine of the Royal College of Anaesthetists, the Royal College of General Practitioners and the Faculty of Addictions of the Royal College of Psychiatrists. January 2010. http://www.britishpainsociety.org/pub_professional.htm#opioids (accessed 7th March 2014).

Optimal Self Care NHS (2005). http://www.brightonandhovepct.nhs.uk (accessed 7th March 2014).

Pain and Self Care Toolkit. http://www.paintoolkit.org/ (accessed 7th March 2014).

Pain Association of Scotland. http://www.painassociation.com (accessed 7th March 2014).

Pain Concern. http://www.painconcern.org.uk (accessed 7th March 2014).

Pain management programmes for adults: information for patients (2007) (PDF) from The British Pain Society Patient publications. http://www.britishpainsociety.org/pub_patient.htm (accessed 7th March 2014).

Pain Relief Foundation. http://www.painrelieffoundation.org.uk (accessed 7th March 2014).

Pain Support. http://www.painsupport.co.uk (accessed 7th March 2014).

Papageorgiou AC *et al.* (2002) Chronic widespread pain in the population: a seven year follow up study. *Ann Rheum Dis* **61:**1071–4.

Patel AS *et al.* (2012) The impact and burden of chronic pain in the workplace: A qualitative systematic review. *Pain Pract* **12:**578–89.

Patient UK for specific pelvic pain information. http://www.patient.co.uk/pils.asp (accessed 7th March 2014).

Pelvic Pain Support Network. http://www.pelvicpain.org.uk (accessed 7th March 2014).

Peul WC *et al.* (2007) Surgery versus prolonged conservative treatment for sciatica. *N Engl J Med* **356:**2245–56.

PharmaGKB: CYP2D6 Dosing Guidelines. http://www.pharmgkb.org/gene/PA128 (accessed 7th March 2014).

Raftery MN *et al.* (2012) The economic cost of chronic noncancer pain in Ireland: Results from the PRIME study, Part 2. *J Pain* **13:**139–45.

Rheumatoid Arthritis Society. http://www.nras.org.uk (accessed 7th March 2014).

Roehrs T and Roth T (2005) Sleep and pain: interaction of two vital functions. *Semin Neurol* **25:**106–16.

Roelofs PDDM *et al.* (2011) Non-steroidal anti-inflammatory drugs for low back pain. Database Syst Rev; CD000396. http://onlinelibrary.wiley.com/doi/10.1002/14651858. CD000396.pub3/pdf/standard (accessed 22 January 2014).

Rooij AD *et al.* (2012) Predictors of multidisciplinary treatment outcome in fibromyalgia: a systematic review. *Disabil Rehabil* **35:**437–49. doi: 10.3109/09638288.2012.699582. Epub 2012 Aug 14.

Rosenstiel AK and Keefe FJ (1983) The use of coping strategies in chronic low back pain patients: relationship to patient characteristics and current adjustment. *Pain* **17:**33–44.

Rossy LA *et al.* (1999) A meta-analysis of fibromyalgia treatment interventions. *Ann Behav Med* **21:**180–91.

Royal College of Psychiatrists report on self-harm, suicide and risk: helping people who self-harm (2010). http://www.rcpsych.ac.uk/files/pdfversion/CR158.pdf (accessed 7th March 2014).

Russell J *et al.* (2000) Efficacy of tramadol in treatment of pain in fibromyalgia. *J Clin Rheumatol* **6:**250–7.

Saarto T and Wiffen PJ (2007) Antidepressants for neuropathic pain, Cochrane Database of Systematic Reviews. Chichester: John Wiley & Sons.

Samaritans. http://www.samaritans.org.uk (accessed 7th March 2014).

Sator-Katzenschlager SM *et al.* (2005) Chronic pelvic pain treated with gabapentin and amitriptyline: A randomized controlled pilot study. *Wiener Klinische Wochenschrift* **117:**761–8.

Scottish Intercollegiate Guidelines Network (2013) SIGN 136: Management of Chronic Pain. NHS Healthcare Improvement Scotland, Edinburgh. http://www.sign. ac.uk/guidelines/fulltext/136/index.html (accessed 19 December 2013).

Scottish legislation on mental capacity. http://bma.org.uk/practical-support-at-work/ ethics/mental-capacity-scotland (accessed 10th May 2012).

Shone N (2002) *Coping with Chronic Pain Successfully*. London: Sheldon Press.

Smith BH and Torrance N (2008) Epidemiology of Chronic Pain. In: *Systematic Reviews in Pain Research: Methodology Refined*. (Eds: McQuay HJ *et al.*) Seattle: IASP Press; pp 247–73.

Smith BH *et al.* (2012) Epidemiology of Back Pain: Time to Research the Role of Biological Mechanisms. In: *From Acute to Chronic Back Pain: Risk Factors, Mechanisms and Clinical Implications*. (Eds: Hasenbring M *et al.*) Oxford: Oxford University Press; pp 3–20.

Smith MT and Haythornthwaite JA (2004) How do sleep disturbance and chronic pain inter-relate? Insights from the longitudinal and cognitive-behavioral clinical trials literature. *Sleep Med Rev* **8:**119–32.

Smith MT *et al.* (2005) Cognitive behavior therapy for chronic insomnia occurring within the context of medical and psychiatric disorders. *Clin Psychol Rev* **25:**559–92.

Spallone V *et al.* (2012) Validation of DN4 as a screening tool for neuropathic pain in painful diabetic polyneuropathy. *Diabet Med* **29:**578–85.

Spitzer RL *et al.* (2006) An ultra-brief scale for anxiety and depression: the GAD-7. *Arch Intern Med* **166:**1092–7.

Sprangers MA *et al.* (2000) Which chronic conditions are associated with better or poorer quality of life? *J Clin Epidemiol* **53:**895–907.

Stanley N (2012) Importance of sleep in neuropathic pain; Bedeutung des Schlafs bei neuropathischen Schmerzen. *Somnologie - Schlafforschung und Schlafmedizin* **16:**17–9.

Statistics on Drug Misuse England 2011. The Health and Social Care Information Centre. http://www.ic.nhs.uk/statistics-and-data-collections/health-and-lifestyles/drug-misuse/statistics-on-drug-misuse-england-2011 (accessed 7th March 2014).

Stiefel F and Stagno D (2004) Management of insomnia in patients with chronic pain conditions. *CNS Drugs* **18:**285–96.

Stones W *et al.* (2005) Interventions for treating chronic pelvic pain in women, Cochrane database of systematic reviews. Chichester: John Wiley & Sons.

Stroke Association. http://www.stroke.org.uk (accessed 7th March 2014).

Talking Health. http://www.talkinghealth.org (accessed 7th March 2014).

Tasman A *et al.* (2008) *Psychiatry*, 3rd edition. Ontario: Wiley & Sons.

Taylor J and Gupta S (2013) The Neurobiology of Persistent Pain: Recent Advances. In: *World Clinics: Anesthesia, Critical Care and Pain*. (Eds: Baheti DK *et al.*) New Dehli: Jaypee Brothers Medical Publishers; pp 1–31.

Teutsch C (2003) Patient-doctor communication. *Med Clin N Am* **87:**1115–45.

The Pain Management Plan. http://www.Npowered.co.uk/ (accessed 7th March 2014).

The Screener and Opioid Assessment for Patients in Pain, revised 2007 (SOAPP-R). http://www.painedu.org/soap.asp (accessed 7th March 2014).

The Patient Experience Review service is designed to support NHS organizations in making the most of their patient experience data. http://www.pickereurope.org/ (accessed 27th September 2012).

Treede RD *et al.* (2008) Neuropathic pain: redefinition and a grading system for clinical and research purposes. *Neurology* **70:**1630–5.

Trigeminal Neuralgia Association UK. http://www.tna-uk.org.uk (accessed 7th March 2014).

Turk DC and Dworkin RH (2004) What should be the core outcomes in chronic pain clinical trials? *Arthritis Res Ther* **6:**151–4.

Turk DC *et al*. (2010) Assessment and treatment of psychosocial comorbidities in patients with neuropathic pain. *Mayo Clin Proc* **85:**S42–50.

United Nations (1948) The Universal Declaration of Human Rights. http://www.un.org/en/documents/udhr/index.shtml#a5 (accessed 11 March 2014).

van Dieen JH *et al*. (2003) Trunk muscle activation in low-back pain patients, an analysis of the literature. *J Electromyogr Kinesiol* **13:**333–51.

Von Korff M *et al*. (1997) Collaborative management of chronic illness *Annals Int Med* **127:**1097–102.

Waddell G (1998) Diagnostic triage. In: *The back pain revolution*. London: Churchill Livingstone; pp 9–25.

Waddell G *et al*. (1980) Non-organic physical signs in low back pain. *Spine* **5:**117–25.

Wang C *et al*. (2010) A randomized trial of tai chi for fibromyalgia. *N Engl J Med* **363:**743–54.

Watson PJ *et al*. (2004) Returning the chronically unemployed with low back pain to employment. *Eur J Pain* **8:**359–69.

White KP *et al*. (2002) Does the label "fibromyalgia" alter health status, function, and health service utilization? A prospective, within-group comparison in a community cohort of adults with chronic widespread pain. *Arthritis & Rheumatism* **47:**260–5.

Whitmore KE (1994) Self-care regimens for patients with interstitial cystitis. *Urol Clin N Am* **21:**121–30.

WHO Suicide Prevention (SUPRE). http://www.who.int/mental_health/prevention/suicide/suicideprevent/en/ (accessed 20th March 2014).

Williams A CdeC and Johnson M (2011) Debate and analysis. Persistent pain: not a medically unexplained symptom. *Brit J Gen Prac* **61:**638–9.

Williams DA (2003) Psychological and behavioural therapies in fibromyalgia and related syndromes. *Best Pract Res Clin Rheumatol* **17:**649–65.

Wilson SJ *et al*. (2010) British Association for Psychopharmacology consensus statement on evidence-based treatment of insomnia, parasomnias and circadian rhythm disorders. *J Psychopharmacol* **24:**1577–601.

Wolfe F *et al*. (1990) The American College of Rheumatology 1990 criteria for the classification of fibromyalgia: report of the multicenter criteria committee. *Arthritis Rheum* **33:**160–72.

Wolfe F *et al*. (2010) The American College of Rheumatology preliminary diagnostic criteria for fibromyalgia and measurement of symptom severity. *Arthritis Care Res (Hoboken)* **62:**600–10.

Your Health Your Way. http://www.nhs.uk/yourhealth (accessed 7th March 2014).